Heal Yourself Naturally Now

With the Established Chinese Technique of *PaidaLajin*

Hongchi Xiao

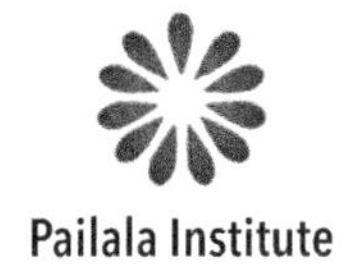
Pailala Institute

Heal Yourself Naturally Now

With the Established, Classic Chinese Technique of *PaidaLajin*
by Hongchi Xiao

Published by

Pailala Institute
17602 17th Street, Suite 102-313
Tustin, CA 92780
Phone: 714-699-3188
Email: team@pailala.org

Translator: Ellen Zhang
Chief Editor: Jen Zelinger
Other Editors: Candida Kutz, Jean Vengua, Lan Ziegler
Book Design: Nick Zelinger

ISBN: 978-1-7320856-0-2 (print)
ISBN: 978-1-7320856-1-9 (eBook)
LCCN: 2018938452

First Edition
Printed in the USA

CONTENTS

Praise for the *Paidalajin* Method

"While researching the Chinese Meridian System on YouTube, I inadvertently stumbled on 'Self-Healing Techniques' in which Master Xiao gave quite a detailed explanation of his philosophy and approach. From prior knowledge and background in natural medicine, I appreciated how and why this therapy works immediately. Such a simple, practical therapeutic application was what I had been hoping to find during my study and practice of natural medicine and also recently, while attempting to recover my own health. The guiding principle that the body has the ability to heal itself underlies many of the modalities used in modern natural medicine. However, Master Xiao's techniques showed me for the very first time how this natural force could be rekindled to extraordinary effect, at the same time covering very broad-spectrum disease.

PaidaLajin Self-healing techniques validates the phrase, 'Nature is the physician of diseases' or 'vix medicatrix naturae', often used in natural medicine and attributed to Hippocrates. The simple techniques demonstrate that, given the right impetus, the human body being the 'living laboratory' that it is, with its innate wisdom, knows exactly how to heal itself. *PaidaLajin*—empiric therapy, yet demonstrably scientific, can only be described as a gift from God.

Master Xiao's *PaidaLajin* self-healing is proof indeed that, 'The natural healing force within each of us is the greatest force in getting well.' And, of course, the phenomenal number of personal experiences and testimonials expressed worldwide speak for themselves. I, too, am pleased to have had the privilege of experiencing its healing effects first-hand."

—Claudia Jane Smith BSc (Hons) Osteopathic Medicine ND DO MRN Registered Naturopathic Physician

"I was born on December 27, 1949 in Jakarta, Indonesia. I studied medicine in Belgium in KUL (Katholieke Universiteit Leuven), where I finished in 1977. In 1979, I passed the examination of medical part of ECFMG (Educational Commission for Medical Graduates) in the USA. From 1980-1985 I followed anaesthesiology training at the O.L.V. (Onze Lieve Vrouw) Clinic in Aalst, Belgium.

I worked as an anesthesiologist in Zuiderzee Hospital in Lelystad, The Netherlands until March 1987. From April 1987 until March 2006, I worked in the Vlietland hospital in Schiedam, the Netherlands. In 1988, I was educated in pain management in the Spaarne hospital by Dr. Michael Sanders, a pain specialist. From 1992-1996, I was a senior lecturer in pain therapy at the Erasmus Medisch Centrum, Rotterdam. In 2000, I passed the examination for x-ray hygiene and became a Fellow of Interventional Pain Practice (FIPP) in 2007.

Between March 2006 and 2016, I worked in the Saint-Anna Hospital in Geldrop, the Netherlands, as a pain practitioner, where I did scientific studies for my PhD thesis with the title: 'Minimally Invasive Therapy in Patients with Head and Neck Pain'.

In my hospital, as a single pain practitioner in 2015, I treated 748 new patients, using radio frequencies, in 1879 cases and other pain treatment techniques in 631 cases.

In 2016, I worked the last year before my retirement and in the last years I thought several times, 'How do I fill my free time? How can I manage my health?'

Herewith, I will tell everybody: I finally learned *PaidaLajin*! It is amazing that I could experience this technique as a relief from what I was suffering from. I got a lot of information about *PaidaLajin* in 2015 from my sister, who is also a doctor (MSc.) But I still ignored this opportunity. The idea to experience *PaidaLajin* came finally in October when I was asked again, after three times, to give a presentation on deep-friction massage. I asked if I could talk about another method. I chose *PaidaLajin* and prepared the presentation. I tried this technique on myself with comfortable, astonishing results for my knees and back. Following this, I advised some patients to do these exercises at home, especially if regular therapy didn't help. On November 27, 2016, I gave a presentation again about *PaidaLajin* to the massage school, Tai Chi school, and my friends. The results are amazing. It increased my motivation and confidence about doing *PaidaLajin*. In 2016, I stopped working as a pain practitioner in Geldrop, The Netherlands. In 2017, I plan to teach at a college at the university in Malang, Indonesia."

—Willy Halim, MD, FIPP

"My name is Dongxiao Zhu. I'm a librarian at Plano Public Library System.

I learned *PaidaLajin* from Master Xiao's Chinese book "Journey to Self-Healing" in 2013 and used this method to heal my frozen shoulder, chronic lower back pain, sharp pain in both knees, tooth pain, sore throat, urinary tract infection ... and the list can go on.

I also used this method to heal my son's stomach pain, my daughter's altitude sickness, my father's difficulty in urination, a friend's tailbone pain, and another friend's high blood pressure.

I've held a bi-weekly *PaidaLajin* meeting at Plano, Texas since June of 2014 and have helped over 100 people in the past three years use and teach this amazing self-healing method.

I strongly recommend Master Xiao's book to anyone who has an open mind and would like to give *PaidaLajin* self-healing a try."

"My name is Lan Ziegler. I live in central PA. I have greatly benefited from the *PaidaLajin* self-healing method—not only lessening and curing my seasonal allergies, lower back pain, and stiff shoulder, and neck pain, but also empowering myself to help other people regain their health and improve their quality of life.

If you are searching for a natural therapy or are tired of swallowing handfuls of prescribed pills every day, please read this book and give it a try. You will be amazed how easy, effective, economic, and eco-friendly this method is.

You will discover our innate self-healing power by awakening it through *PaidaLajin*, one of the ancient Chinese health practices."

—email: dadaozhijianpaila@gmail.com

The Five-Minute Diagnosis

Would you be interested in taking five minutes to discover if you have blocked circulation?

According to Traditional Chinese Medicine, the cause of most disease is microcirculation blockages: the last path of exchanged nutrients and toxins through your capillaries and the lymph nodes connected to your organs.

In all of Mr. Xiao's seminars, he begins clearing these blockages by having everyone slap the inner elbow of their left arm for five minutes.

He says, "You can tolerate five minutes of pain, can't you? Don't worry, you will not feel pain after three minutes. We guarantee it."

90% of people show some purple or black marks during the process: a sign of blockages to the Heart Meridian—and most people feel pain.

Many people assume these marks are bruises (broken blood vessels). If you worry about that, try slapping the middle of your forearm. You will notice that no matter how hard you slap, no color (outside of some temporary reddening) will ever last. This is because blockages always occur at places we bend or at the tip of our limbs.

These colored spots are exactly the same as the purple marks on Michael Phelps shoulders. You may have seen them during the Olympics. They are the toxins in his body, blocking his microcirculation, coming to the surface.

Make sure you slap hard enough, but not too quickly. Slap for about half a second each time. The more pain you feel, the more blocked the region is.

It sounds counterintuitive, but slap even harder.

After three minutes, no one feels pain anymore.

During the fourth and fifth minutes, slap even harder.

If you are familiar with Chinese meridian charts, you can try a more academic test:

Find a spot on your body that appears to bruise after you slap it for a minute. You might need to try a number of spots before you find one that does more than turn red.

After you discover the spot, try two things.

First of all, continue to slap the spot until the color disappears. Remember, it may seem like a bruise, but if you continue to slap the area, it will disappear. After that happens for the first time, you will gain trust in the method.

After that, look up which energetic meridians run through that part of your body online, especially if it took a long time to make the color disappear or if it also became swollen. Chances are very likely that the acupressure point you found will be related to a health concern you have—or have had in the past.

But don't look it up until after you've tested the method!

INTRODUCTION

Can I Really Heal Myself?

The medical industry wastes enormous financial resources on the downstream of life, trying to solve health problems instead of preventing them. Doctors rescue "drowning" patients, while ignoring soil and water conservation in the upper reaches of the river.

Instead of repeating the same old story, can humanity solve problems—earlier rather than later?

This book provides both a philosophy and a method to achieve that goal: *PaidaLajin*, a method to activate the self-healing mechanisms within us.

Unlike medical therapy options, *PaidaLajin* embraces muscular exercises simpler than yoga and *t'ai chi*. Almost anyone, of any age, can learn the techniques in a few minutes. *PaidaLajin* reclaims our human nature—and manifests the divine within us.

Thanks to its simple and effective nature *PaidaLajin*:

- Spread to over sixty countries and territories over the past six years.
- Aided tens of millions of people with different skin colors, religious beliefs, and social backgrounds.
- Received testimonials from people across the world.

The original edition of this book, in Chinese, sold over a million copies.

Our data, collected from 2009–2015, conservatively estimates *PaidaLajin* helps prevent or heal 50% of all illnesses. These include:

- Chronic pain
- Cancer

- Stroke
- Diabetes
- Psoriasis
- Depression
- Hypertension
- Heart disease
- Uterine fibroids
- Type I and II diabetes
- Hypertension
- Heart disease
- Parkinson's disease
- Conditions recognized by Chinese Medicine

In August 2011, we followed up with telephone interviews after workshops in China. We discovered:

1. *PaidaLajin* was 86% effective in assisting people with diabetes, hypertension, lower back pain, and leg pain.
2. 93% of participants reported better health, compared to taking medications for the same conditions.
3. The remaining 7% maintained the same health as when medicated—without the medication!

In 2015, we conducted a 5-day-workshop with the TAG VHS Diabetes Research Centre in India, strictly complying with requirements similar to Western medical research.

The medical experts' clinical report evidenced *PaidaLajin* can indeed improve health, enthusiasm, and energy levels. It demonstrated a curative effect on chronic diseases, and an even higher recorded value when eliminating pain.

In December 2015, other surveys showed a 90% improvement in diabetes, hypertension, and heart disease. This was also true for neck, shoulder, back, waist, and leg pain. Whether or not they continued to practice *PaidaLajin* at home after the workshop, participant's conditions improved. The 84% who continued the practice experienced the most obvious improvements. Over 62% discontinued medication (with physician approval.)

PaidaLajin relieves acute heart attacks more effectively than cardiopulmonary resuscitation (CPR.) It helps with non-bleeding acute symptoms, such as cold, fever, cramps, headaches, motion sickness, menstrual pain, acute gastroenteritis, acute heart attack, and acute sports injuries—at a rate of 80%.

The creators of *PaidaLajin* derived it from an ancient outlook on the universe and healthcare: positive energy wards off illness, traceable back to the ancient Chinese classics, *The Huang Di Nei Jing* (*The Yellow Emperor's Canon of Internal Medicine*) and *The Tao Te Ching*. Everyone who supports *PaidaLajin* has one thing in common: they personally practice it

In addition to *PaidaLajin*, we recommend practicing Heart Chan Meditation, based on the same principles. We invited well-seasoned meditation teacher Donald Hwong to teach participants at a *PaidaLajin* workshop in California. Those with experience found *PaidaLajin* helped them meditate more easily and deeply; those with no previous meditation experienced a cleansing of their blocked meridians.

During our workshops, we meditate twice a day—once in the morning and once in the evening. Both *PaidaLajin* and meditation modes for internal cleansing, based on the same traditional Chinese Medicine principles. *PaidaLajin* focuses on physical healing, while Heart Chan Meditation eliminates worries, fears, and resentment: the major causes of all illness.

Our body, heart, and soul are an integral whole. Improving our physical health naturally enhances the quality of meditation, leading to spiritual ascension.

The universe provides the options, but human beings have abandoned them. However, these capabilities exist within human culture, like an ancient seed, lying dormant for millennia. It's waiting to surface: our innate, self-healing mechanism. Humans are the only species on Earth that forfeited self-healing, while plants and animals maintain it.

I included a link to the Heart Chan Meditation book on the final page. We hope readers will combine both to enjoy a holistic, joyful life experience.

PaidaLajin is like driving a car; the hardware and software is already there. We only need to use a key to start the engine

Hongchi Xiao
February 5, 2016

DEDICATION and ACKNOWLEDGMENTS

This work is dedicated to my family, friends, volunteers, and team members who have been supportive all along, particularly during tough times, and to people across the world who are open to the idea of self-healing through *PaidaLajin*.

My special thanks go to Ellen Zhang, who helped edit the Chinese manuscript and translated it into English.

- Translator: Ellen Zhang
- Editors: Jen Zelinger, Candida Kutz, Jean Vengua, and Lan Ziegler

I also like to express my gratitude to all the teachers who taught me about Traditional Chinese Medicine, as well as the dedicated research done by Dr. Alfred Pischinger on matrix biology. Without them, I would not have recognized the power of self-healing through *PaidaLajin* or realized that *PaidaLajin* can be explained scientifically.

After so many years of hearing thousands of new testimonials and new cases that *PaidaLajin* has healed, I have recently come to realize that such an intricate design of the human body, and the gift of self-healing, can only be manifested by God. He continuously surprises me, giving me amazing insight into our world. Thank you, God.

MEDICAL DISCLAIMER

This book describes self-healing exercises.

PaidaLajin includes slapping and stretching exercises available to everyone—similar to yoga and t'ai chi. They are not a medical treatment. Those who practice *PaidaLajin* and believe in self-healing benefit enormously.

The statements in this book have not been evaluated by the FDA. Self-healing with *PaidaLajin* is not intended to be a substitute for professional medical advice, diagnosis, or treatment. Always seek the advice of your physician or other qualified health care providers with any questions you may have regarding a medical condition. Never disregard professional medical advice or delay in seeking it because of the information provided herein.

This publication contains the opinions and witnesses of its author. It is intended to provide helpful and informative material on the subject matter covered. The author and publisher specifically disclaim any responsibility for any liability, loss, or risk (personal or otherwise) that is incurred as a consequence, directly or indirectly, of the use and application of any of the contents of this book.

1

THE THEORY AND HISTORY OF *PAIDALAJIN*

What is Self-Healing?

Humans, animals, and plants have the inherent ability to repair and heal themselves. Any method that mobilizes this power is self-healing.

Building up our immune system, which fights disease, is a large part of our self-healing power. It enables the body to produce a variety of biochemical substances that address a person's specific needs. These biochemical substances can be referred to as endogenous (or organic) medicine. They don't have side effects.

Hippocrates, the Father of Western Medicine, repeatedly stressed that the body possesses the power to balance and heal itself. It is the duty of a medical practitioner to tap into this power: an ancient interpretation of self-healing.

Seven Requirements for Self-Healing

People have practiced yoga, judo, dance, kungfu, *qi gong*, aerobics, *taekwondo, t'ai chi*, other sports, and meditation throughout human history, as methods of self-healing. We promote the teachings in *Huang Di Nei Jing* (simplified Chinese: 黄帝内经; traditional Chinese: 黃帝內經; *pinyin*: *huáng dì nèi jīng*), also known as *The Yellow Emperor's Canon of Internal Medicine*, an ancient Chinese medical book. For two thousand years, it has been considered the foundational resource for Chinese Medicine.

Huang Di Nei Jing advocates these steps:

1. Nurse the Heart.
2. Use natural and dietary therapy methods.
3. Use medication as a last resort.

(Note: "heart" refers to the physical organ. "Heart" refers to the big picture of human emotions.)

How do we nurse the heart?

We need a simple system without side effects. Over the years, my search for traditional healing has taken me on many journeys. Through education and repeated practice, I found simple and effective methods. I summed up seven criteria to determine whether a healing method will be readily embraced and beneficial.

1. **Do It Yourself**
   Everyone should have access to self-help exercises for health.
2. **Effective**
   Its effectiveness should be equivalent or superior to mainstream medicine.
3. **Simple**
   People should be able to learn the techniques in a few minutes.
4. **Safe**
   It should have no side effects.
5. **Comprehensive**
   It should effectively address most physical and mental disorders, including common, acute, chronic, critical, and rare diseases.
6. **Low-Cost or Free**
   It should be available to everyone, despite income. Our goal is to save enormous medical expenses for individuals, families, organizations, and nations.

7. **Organic**
   It shouldn't rely on additional medicine or treatment.

At first glance, it seems impossible to meet the criteria on this list.

Fortunately, we found such methods, and we have been teaching them across the world. They are *Paida* and *Lajin*: slapping and stretching exercises. We'll refer to them as *PaidaLajin* from now on.

They are not my inventions, but folk secret therapies, practiced in China for millennia, including in the *Huang Di Nei Jing* and *The Tao Te Ching*. In fact, different variations of slapping and stretching exercises can be found throughout the ages and around the world. You've clapped your hands and stretched your limbs, haven't you?

Promoting secret healing therapies is challenging, especially with legal restrictions. Fortunately, the internet gives millions of people access to information. Anyone can practice and test *PaidaLajin*.

What is *PaidaLajin*?

Paida involves using our hands or tools to repeatedly slap parts of our bodies to a degree we can tolerate.

It helps the natural energy in our body flow through the meridians, which are areas in the body connected to specific organs. It can be practiced by yourself or with others. *Paida* is a natural diagnostic method, used to discover which parts of our bodies are sick. In ancient times, *Paida* was called *diao shang* (revealing old injuries.)

During *Lajin*, we stretch our limbs and joints to set our bones correctly. It also keeps our tendons flexible to assist with the flow of energy in the meridians.

Practicing *PaidaLajin* boosts *qi* (vital life energy) and blood flow. We may initially feel discomfort at the blockages, including pain, soreness, numbness, and swelling at the sites. This is due to the toxins and wastes that induced the disease in first place.

Increasing *qi*:

- Helps with diagnosing diseases
- Treats the conditions
- Prevents further disease
- Stimulates immune responses
- Reduces the effects of aging, increasing life expectancy

PaidaLajin's efficacy has been scientifically measured in addressing:

- Pain
- Diabetes
- Hypertension
- Heart disease
- Parkinson's disease

They are also based on the testimonials from millions of people who practice it.

The advantages of *PaidaLajin*:

- It's accessible to everyone
- The effects are obvious
- It can easily be shared with others

Ironically, *PaidaLajin's* amazing healing effects can also be a drawback: it seems too good to be true. We are used to complexity in healing, so simple treatments contradict mainstream education. Self-healing with *PaidaLajin* involves adapting your mind and way of life, which is a great challenge for many people.

Everyone who formally supports self-healing with *PaidaLajin* have one thing in common: they came to their conclusions after personal practice.

The truest way is also the simplest. Practice *PaidaLajin* yourself, and you will learn the benefits.

2

THE MAIN CONCEPTS OF *PAIDALAJIN*

Ignore the Name of the Disease

This is the primary concept behind *PaidaLajin*, and the secret to successful self-healing.

Someone who is new to *PaidaLajin* might ask, "Where do I slap to heal heart disease?" In order to benefit from the treatment, you have to let go of the idea of a specific illness and focus on your body as a whole. If you do *PaidaLajin* systematically, you will heal your entire body—and keep it healthy!

There are problems with focusing on a specific disease. You likely suffer from other underlying diseases the doctors aren't aware of. We've learned to label diseases in modern medicine based on pathological indicators and statistics, but these labels may not address the underlying causes. Dispensing prescriptions based solely on a diagnosed disease—with no regard to causes—may worsen conditions.

Disease names can be very misleading. I will use two very common ones, diabetes and hypertension, to exemplify my point.

Diabetes Type II

A diabetes diagnosis misleadingly focuses on blood glucose levels.

After you're diagnosed, you begin hypoglycemic drugs to control your blood sugar. However, the medication can lead to glaucoma—or even heart problems.

In addition to causing further health issues, this approaches the cause of diabetes incorrectly. When practicing *PaidaLajin*, people exhibiting diabetes discover *sha*, a colorful toxic waste that appears during *Paida*, when the inner elbows are slapped.

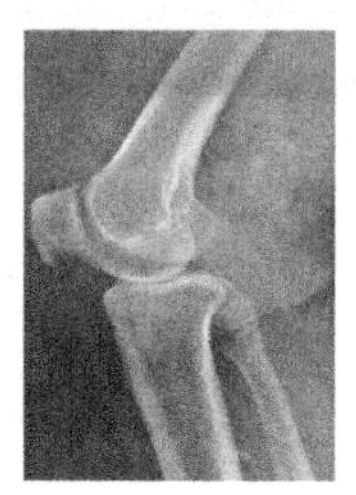

The Heart and Pericardium Meridians run along the inner elbows. This signals a person already has undiagnosed heart problems. If these people practice *Lajin* in Reclining Posture, they feel pain at the root of their thighs and the back of their knees. This pain indicates the Liver, Spleen, Kidney, and Urinary Bladder Meridians are all blocked, so the corresponding organs are ill. Problems in these organs are the underlying cause of diabetes.

Further investigation reveals all diabetics suffer from emotional disorders to varying degrees, such as tension, anxiety, and depression. Such emotional turmoil leads to endocrine disorders. Most teenaged students are stressed out before sitting for a major exam. If tested, they exhibit endocrine disorders and abnormal blood glucose levels.

In short, diabetes is caused by endocrine disorders, related to the Heart. Since we define the Heart as the big picture of human emotion, diabetes is—at its core—an emotional problem. When people are obsessed with money, power, or social status, they become tense and anxious. This stress leads many people to eat and drink too much, causing endocrine system malfunctions.

Taking hypoglycemic drugs causes further damage to the heart, liver, kidneys, spleen, and pancreas—making the problems worse, not better.

According to Chinese Medicine, the Liver Meridian connects to the eyes. As long as the liver functions normally, the eyes will be healthy. Hypoglycemic drugs and injecting insulin damages the liver, leading to eye problems, such as glaucoma and retinal detachment. Many diabetics on medication end up with eye and internal organ problems. When the condition worsens, their feet will ulcerate, even to a degree that requires amputation.

To cure diabetes, we must not be misled by its name. We need to identify the real causes. Diabetics should first be happy and self-assured—and learn to let go of stress. Practicing *PaidaLajin* unblocks the Heart, Liver, Spleen, Kidney, and Urinary Bladder Meridians. When the internal organs function well, the blood glucose level will normalize.

Hypertension

Anti-hypertensive drugs are often used to control blood pressure. However, these drugs often damage the heart, liver, spleen, kidneys, and other organs.

Almost all antihypertensive drugs are diuretics, designed to increase the amount of water and salt expelled from the body. They weaken the functions of the kidneys, potentially leading to:

- Lower libido
- Decline of sexual function
- Prostate disorders
- Frequent and involuntary urination
- Insomnia
- Tinnitus

- Hearing loss
- Hair loss
- Bone loss
- Alzheimer's disease
- A shortened lifespan

The acidity of the medications can also destroy the tissues of blood vessel walls, causing strokes and heart disease.

It is clearly stated in the Chinese medical classic *Huang Di Nei Jing* that "The Kidney governs the bones; its health is shown in the hair; it opens into the ears; and it controls memory, the urinary and excretory functions, and governs natural lifespan."

Blood pressure will return to normal when the Heart, Liver, Spleen and Kidney Meridians are clear.

In effect, there is no definitive standard for normal blood pressure; it relates to a person's age, physique, and many other factors. It changes from day to day, and it fluctuates with the person's mood and activities. Antihypertensive drugs inevitably induce more disorders, including:

- Eye disorders
- Liver disease
- Kidney malfunctions
- Stomach problems

Even more drugs are needed to treat these new diseases. Many hypertensive patients die after years of medication, yet their deaths are not caused by high blood pressure. In this sense, the name hypertension is quite misleading.

We advocate ignoring the name of the disease to remind you there are many root causes behind one particularly labeled disease. The names diabetes and hypertension imply symptoms, not causes. This phenomenon is referred to as complex diseases. All diseases are complex diseases.

A disease indicates various causes for blocked meridians. We want to unblock all of our meridians to achieve optimal health. In fact, the only real healing is holistic healing. Targeting a particular disease or body part, while ignoring the whole, always invites endless trouble. *PaidaLajin* should be practiced on all parts of the body in a carpet-bombing manner to activate our internal anti-virus mechanism. It will clear the body of all disease.

Complex Diseases

People seldom suffer from one illness. Diseases and symptoms are interrelated.

In effect, all diseases are complex. Even such common ailments as colds, fevers, and coughs are complex diseases. They relate to the immune system, which is in turn relates to the heart, lungs, liver, spleen, and kidneys. Chronic diseases such as diabetes, heart disease, hypertension, liver and kidney disorders, and cancer are—without a doubt—complex diseases. They are manifestations of the malfunction of all internal organs.

Since diseases are invariably complex, we need to turn our attention to the underlying causes and holistically empower our self-healing mechanism to do its job. Self-healing power, above all else, cures sickness. Holistic healing goes beyond compartmentalized treatments and addresses all cells, organs, and systems in our body as an integral whole. They thrive or wither together.

No therapy or drug in the world is a panacea. There are many natural, holistic therapies out there. We chose *Paida* and *Lajin* to promote worldwide for the reasons we've noted, but also because they do not target a specific disease or symptom. Rather, they activate *qi*, which empowers the body to clear its own energetic blocks. From diagnosis to treatment, *Paida* and *Lajin* function holistically. This explains why they are so effective in healing complex, chronic diseases.

The fundamental cause of complex diseases is meridian blockage. Unblocking the blockages heals. The beauty of *Paida* and *Lajin* is they rapidly and effectively unblock the obstructions in the meridian system (a network of energy channels.)

Many people know the benefits of acupoints, also known as acupuncture points. They are locations along meridians you stimulate for disease prevention, diagnosis, and treatment. However, it may be hard to find acupoints, since they require complicated knowledge, drugs, equipment, and procedures—that is why many people give up on self-healing their meridians. For ordinary people, without specialized training, *PaidaLajin* is the best basic healing practice. It can also be an advanced therapy if you dig deeper and find its full potential.

Efficacy is what really matters. *Paida* and *Lajin* may appear simple, but they can be more effectual than mainstream medical practices. Many diseases doctors can't cure are self-healed by ordinary people, using these two unbelievably simple methods. The truest way is the simplest: this is an accurate and concrete interpretation of The *Tao* (The Way.)

People gain fresh insights into life and health when they self-heal complex diseases. You will improve your quality of life, thanks to your improved health condition. You will move from physical healing to spiritual healing, and from health management to life management.

Carpet Bombing and the Anti-Virus Mechanism

Originally a military term, carpet bombing refers to thoroughly bombing each and every inch of a target. Practicing *PaidaLajin* in a carpet-bombing manner—slapping the entire body from head to toe, while stretching in Reclining Posture, gradually stretching each leg for up to thirty minutes—clears the body's fourteen main meridians.

In *Paida*, *sha*, swelling, and pain are positive reactions, indicating meridians running along the slapped areas are blocked. It is evidence detoxification is in process. Those afraid of *sha*, swelling, and pain mistake the rewards for punishment. In *Lajin*, the pain during stretching indicates contraction of tendons, ligaments, and blockages in meridians. Continued stretching restores the flexibility of tendons and ligaments, clears the meridians, and heals diseases.

Our body has an invisible anti-virus mechanism, akin to a computer's anti-virus software. The meridian system in Chinese Medicine, and related systems in Western Medicine, such as the immune, nervous, respiratory, and circulatory systems, are all parts of the body's virus-fighting system.

The invisible can be more crucial than the visible. For instance, the sun and the moon are visible, but the orbits they travel and the forces that drive them are invisible. Chinese Medicine asserts *qi* propels blood flow. Blood is visible, whereas *qi*—the driving force behind blood flow—is invisible to the naked eye. Modern scientific devices have detected the invisible *qi* and meridians in the human body.

The wisdom, sensitivity, and sophistication of man's self-healing power go beyond our knowledge and imagination. Even the best scientists and medical professionals have just scratched the surface of this power. Once the anti-virus mechanism is activated through *PaidaLajin*, it will scan the entire body. When *qi* finds a blockage or a problem area, it will lock-in on the target. This process is similar to launching missiles in precision bombing or GPS precise-point positioning.

The carpet bombing isn't localized. It's generalized to all known and unknown systems of the body. The activated *qi* and blood flow not only detect viruses, they stimulate the body to produce antibodies against them. Practicing *PaidaLajin* is like an all-round mobilization of software and hardware systems in the body. This is why it is described as a "complete virus removal".

PaidaLajin dredges meridians. Once blockages are removed, *qi* and blood will flow normally. Moreover, by practicing *PaidaLajin*, *yang* energy rises and *yin* energy falls. Here, *yang* (simplified Chinese: 阳; traditional Chinese: 陽; *pinyin*: *yáng*) is the same as the character in the Chinese words for the sun—*tai yang* (simplified Chinese: 太阳; traditional Chinese: 太陽; *pinyin*: *tài yang*.) It is the original energy in the universe; it is the *zheng-qi* described in *Huang Di Nei Jing*; it is the first breath of air blown into man according to Genesis in the Old Testament of the Bible. It plays a vital role in a person's health.

According to *Huang Di Nei Jing*, the way to maintain good health is to: "Keep *zheng-qi* (positive *yang* energy) inside, and evil shall not enter." It sums up the true essence of healing in Chinese Medicine.

The minimal, self-inflicted damage produced by *PaidaLajin* stimulates the body's immune system to secrete stem cells, insulin, enkephalin, adrenaline, and other hormones needed to fight disease.

The Urinary Bladder Meridian normally hurts the most when stretching on a *Lajin* bench, because an important acupoint is located behind each knee. It's easily blocked and quite painful when stimulated. The Urinary Bladder Meridian runs from head to toe, making it the largest detoxification channel in our body. Cleaning this meridian cures numerous health issues, such as:

- Lower back and leg pain
- Diabetes
- Hypertension
- Heart disease
- Liver problems
- Kidney disorders
- Prostate disorders
- Gynecological disorders
- Cancer

The Urinary Bladder Meridian links the head, neck, back, waist, and legs. It connects to all of the internal organs hanging inside the torso along the spine and forms a web of meridians along with the Spleen, Liver, and Kidney Meridians. It connects to other main meridians as well.

When stretching on a *Lajin* bench, some people can't straighten their raised leg or lower it to touch the ground. They feel excruciating pain while stretching. This indicates problems with the Urinary Bladder, Liver, Spleen, and Kidney Meridians, and it impacts all internal organs. There are three *yin* meridians: the Liver, Spleen, and Kidney Meridians along the inner side of each leg. Once these three meridians are cleared of blockages, diabetes, hypertension, prostate, and gynecological disorders will cease to exist.

Some people like to slap along the Gall Bladder Meridian on the outer side of each leg. It is equally important to slap the inner side. Elderly men who suffer from prostate disorders whose main symptoms are urgent, frequent, and incomplete urination benefit most from doing this in the reclining position. Over 90% of elderly men suffer from prostate problems. For a woman, slapping the inner side of the legs while in Reclining Posture helps relieve almost all gynecological disorders.

The carpet bombing approach to *Paida* results in a more thorough detoxification. For instance, slapping all around the limbs—focusing on one region until *sha* appears and continuing *Paida* until *sha* disappears—is even better. Slapping thoroughly from head to toe, including the head, neck, face, eyes, ears, nose, mouth, breasts, armpits, belly, groin, buttocks, back, and entire spine brings about remarkable healing effects.

Why is this "software" so powerful? Because it is not man-made—it is designed and embedded in us by the universe.

Pain and "Pain Medicine"

Joy without pain is not true happiness. In Chinese, the characters 痛 (pain) and 快 (joy) are put together to form a phrase 痛快 (pain and joy.)

Indeed, pain and joy are two sides of the same coin. There is some pain during *PaidaLajin*, but it's manageable. If you are afraid of pain, the solution is simple: just reduce the intensity of *PaidaLajin*.

Nobody likes pain, but it is ultimately a gift to us. The pain here isn't similar to injuries or accidents. It comes from voluntary practice.

Pain is precisely why we practice *PaidaLajin*. The logic of self-healing with *PaidaLajin* goes like this: the more pain you feel during the practice, the more necessary it is for you to practice it. Once you heal your energetic meridians, the pain immediately disappears.

Pain is a Health Alarm

Pain is a very accurate diagnostic method. According to Chinese Medicine, "No blockage, no pain." The more pain felt during *PaidaLajin*, the more severe the problem. If there is pain along a meridian, it indicates problems with the corresponding organ. For instance, when you have a heart disease and problems with the intangible Heart, the Heart and Pericardium Meridians must be blocked. Slapping these meridians, on the inner elbows, will cause pain and *sha*.

PaidaLajin does not induce pain; rather, pain already lurks inside the body. Imagine it's a hidden bomb—it could explode at any moment.

To avoid the explosion, we practice *PaidaLajin* to bring the latent bombs to the surface and gradually clear them away. People with smoothly flowing meridians do not face the threat. When they practice *PaidaLajin*, they feel little or no pain.

In other words, you can't avoid pain by not practicing *PaidaLajin*. As long as you have a health problem, the pain exists like a time bomb and will most likely worsen—exploding when you least expect it. For instance, a sudden heart attack, stroke, or cancer diagnosis are eventual outbreaks.

The sooner you practice *PaidaLajin*, the earlier you sound the health alarm. If you avoid or cover up pain with anaesthetics, the situation becomes more dangerous. You have removed the health alarm. Very ill patients are more afraid of pain than well people, due to more severe meridian blockages. Hence, the intensity of pain reflects the severity of a disease.

Experiencing Pain is Related to Self-Healing

According to Chinese Medicine, pain during *PaidaLajin* is the process of *yang* energy rising. It produces medicine in vivo (within the living.) Persistent pain indicates continuous production of the medicine.

Pain directly stimulates and opens up the Heart, triggers willpower, and mobilizes *yang* energy. The Heart, King of Internal Organs, governs the spirit. Although pain can be felt all over the body, it is the Heart that feels pain first. It mobilizes the body's resources to deal with the crisis. *Qi* and blood flow most rapidly to the problem area, in an attempt to protect the body.

According to Western Medicine, pain stimulates the endocrine system to secrete biochemical substances the body needs. Endogenous medicine means a treatment the body creates for itself. These include, but are not limited to, various hormones and stem cells. Pain is a natural response to the creation of these factors.

Perhaps pain, itself, is the medicine.

We are educated to regard pain as something negative—even evil—and try our best to avoid it. Seen from another perspective, pain and illness are good—they are warning signs that point us in the direction of healing.

This Pain Medicine Accurately Pinpoints the Location of Diseases

Pain accurately reveals the targets, and persistent pain requires continuous treatment.

When healing is manifested in this way, compared with medication, it is more accurate, symptom-free, and eco-friendly. People feel pain in different parts of their bodies. The intensity differs, so the target and dose differ accordingly.

In Chinese Medicine, self-healing power is referred to as *yang* energy. In Western Medicine, it is referred to as insulin, endorphins, adrenaline, enkephalin, stem cells, immunity, and self-repair ability, among other terms. With the advancement of medical science, new terms will continually join the list.

The Intensity of Pain is Proportionate to the Efficacy of the Treatment

In other words: the more it hurts, the more it heals.

During *PaidaLajin*, when *yang* energy rises faster, you feel more pain. Hormonal changes occur more rapidly. Your entire body warms up and begins to sweat.

The pain of *PaidaLajin* is bearable, and it can be self-regulated according to the person's condition and tolerance. If the pain is almost unbearable, the intensity of *PaidaLajin* should be reduced.

It is impossible for different people to compare the pain of *PaidaLajin*, for the severity of each person's meridian blockages are different. When slapping the same body part on different people, patients who are more ill will tend to feel greater pain.

According to Western Medicine, detoxification and healing happen when the body decomposes and excretes unwanted biochemical substances, producing what the body needs in its place.

According to Chinese Medicine, the *qi* of diseases is *yin* energy. When it accumulates, more diseases will break out and life is shortened. By contrast, when *yang* energy is abundant, fewer diseases will strike and life is prolonged.

Pain is a Method of Meditation and Enhancing Attention

During meditation, you may find it hard to concentrate—your Heart is not at peace and your mind is filled with too many thoughts.

When you feel pain during *PaidaLajin*, your mind is more focused than ever. It is impossible to think about the things that normally occupy your mind. Your attention is focused on the parts that hurt the most. The ability to endure pain fluctuates with changing states of mind, and it is enhanced by continued *PaidaLajin*. The pain becomes a bridge, linking your body, mind, and soul, which continually interact when you feel pain. Pain forces you to focus, which enables you to experience the state of your body, mind, and soul becoming one—the act is both giving and receiving.

Pain Medicine is Essentially Medicine for the Heart

Pain stimulates the Heart, forcing it to adapt or change. It is the result of an interaction between the body and the mind. While pain is felt during *PaidaLajin*, disease is revealed as visible *sha* and swelling appears. Past memories and negative feelings surface. They can then be released. As a result, *PaidaLajin* is great for healing depression and other psychological disorders.

Once you change your mindset and view pain as a positive experience, you can instantly endure greater pain. It will no longer be an enemy, but rather a friend and a teacher. However, if you have negative feelings about the pain, your tolerance will be weakened, and the pain medicine will be less effective.

PaidaLajin Will Enhance Your Pain Tolerance

When you have better resistance to the pain medicine of *PaidaLajin*, it indicates your condition is improving. You will eventually be cured. Once your resistance to externally produced medicine gets stronger, it implies the medicine has become ineffective.

Pain is internal and intangible. *PaidaLajin* is safer and more organic than pills. When it exceeds your endurance, you will instinctively stop taking it by reducing the intensity and length of the sessions. The pain can be managed, according to your needs.

Beginners, the elderly, and the seriously ill shouldn't start *PaidaLajin* with high intensity. They should begin slowly and patiently await results.

A Warm Body Reduces Pain

Qi and blood flow faster after bathing in a hot spring, a footbath, a warm-water shower, or a sauna. If you practice *PaidaLajin* then, the pain will be less intense, and *sha* will appear and disappear faster.

Healing Reactions

Healing reactions, also known as detox reactions, flare reactions, or healing crises are typical during *PaidaLajin*. They are inevitable. You are allowing illness to surface and be healed, rather than suppressing it and covering it up. It is a dialogue between the body, mind, and soul—not a life-or-death war.

Once *PaidaLajin* activates the self-healing power within us, this power will start to scan the entire body and dredge all blockages.

Various reactions occur during this process. Possible side effects include:

Hot and cold flashes, soreness, numbness, itching, pain, swelling, rashes, sweating, nausea, vomiting, diarrhea, dry mouth, bloating, stomachaches, dizziness, or drowsiness. Black or purple *sha*, red swellings, and greenish bruises (differing forms of *sha*) may appear at the slapped areas.

These are healing reactions (healing crises) intertwined with danger and opportunity. They are similar to those experienced during medication use, acupressure, acupuncture, moxibustion, skin-scraping, cupping therapy, *qi gong*, meditation, and other natural therapies. They are normal physiological reactions when boosted *yang* energy fights *yin* energy that lurks in the body. The *yin*-blocked areas are the source of the problems.

When the boosted *yang* energy tries to go through the blockages, there is greater pressure at these areas. The body manifests various symptoms, similar to those you feel when sick. Healing reactions can end on the same day or they may also last for days, or even weeks, depending on each individual's physique and health condition. Many people are unaware these symptoms are great signs of recovery. They can become frightened. Unfortunately, they may stop *PaidaLajin* entirely.

When healing occurs, various excretions may be expelled from the body in the form of sweat, tears, rashes, vomit, burps, wind, urine, stool, and nasal discharge. These are all good signs detoxification is in process. When Wang Fengyi (1864–1937), a revered Chinese healer who cured patients for free, told patients the root causes of their diseases were wrong thoughts and behaviors, the gravely ill ones often reacted with crying and vomiting. Some people vomited for a long time, even for days on end. It sounds frightening, but the result was gradual recoveries.

In short, healing reactions may appear unpleasant, but they are actually signs of improvement. They are gifts from nature, just like darkness before dawn and pain during childbirth.

Testimonials About Healing Reactions

You can find these real-life testimonials of ordinary people dealing with healing reactions by visiting http://pailala.org.

Self-Diagnosis

The philosophy of self-healing of *PaidaLajin* is contrary to mainstream medicine. It enables the body to reveal its own health problems. By contrast, medication and surgery tend to cover them up.

Symptoms show us which parts of the body are sick. They include agonies we suffer from, illnesses and injuries from the past, and diseases that are yet to express themselves.

Paida was once called *diao shang* (revealing diseases and injuries.) The first step of self-healing is to dig up all illnesses, particularly hidden symptoms, and allow them to go away or change their nature.

PaidaLajin puts into practice the philosophy of action through inaction, advocated in the Chinese ancient classic *The Tao Te Ching.* It follows natural law—The *Tao*—the way the universe, nature, and matter work. Various health problems surface, and the real causes are detected.

Antibiotics kill bacteria, painkillers "kill" pain, sleeping pills cover up insomnia, antihypertensive drugs lower blood pressure, hypoglycemic drugs control blood sugar, chemotherapy kills cancer cells, and surgery removes tumors.

Attention is focused on eliminating symptoms, while their causes remains, waiting to create future problems.

Action through inaction means following The *Tao* and only doing simple, necessary things.

PaidaLajin uses simple methods to cure us naturally, without our intervention. *Paida* reveals and heals past injuries and diseases we may think we've left behind. Some people call it *da gui* (beating the demons), because it drives evil energy out of the body. In cases where diseases go undetected or are misdiagnosed, *PaidaLajin* can immediately fix the diagnosis.

The Body Protects and Heals Itself

PaidaLajin might yield immediate results, but it is more likely to take some time and result in temporary side effects. The symptoms will surface, and sometimes even worsen, before they are fixed. It is like playing a cat-and-mouse game. In addition to soreness, numbness, itching, pain, and swelling, there may also be tears, rashes, red spots, dizziness, headaches, insomnia, coughing, belching, nausea, vomiting, thick phlegm, a runny nose, watery or bloody blisters, flatulence, or smelly urine and stool. These are signs of the body expelling toxic waste. These toxins come from years of accumulated negative feelings, cigarettes, medication, and injections as well as air, food, and water pollution. The smell of drugs and cigarettes can come out through skin pores and other bodily orifices, even decades after their intake. If your Kidney and Urinary Bladder Meridians are blocked, your urine might turn red, brown, or black.

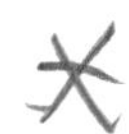

Clinical results continually prove that the more severe the healing reactions, the better the self-healing effects.

More severe healing reactions include cramps all over the body or even fainting, similar to responses to acupuncture treatments. Past illnesses may surface and worsen during *PaidaLajin*:

- Cardiovascular patients may feel more heart discomfort
- Hypertensive patients may have higher blood pressure
- Diabetics might have higher blood glucose levels
- Patients with gastric problems may experience more stomach discomfort
- Pain may intensify

This healing crises indicate the positive and negative energies are engaged in a fight. According to Chinese Medicine, when *yin* and *yang* energies are balanced, pain and disease are healed. According to Western Medicine, the body is:

- Producing useful hormones and stem cells
- Discharging harmful hormones
- Disposing of malfunctioning and dead cells

Do not assume these intense reactions are bad. These rewards are not punishments. The best thing to do at this point is continue *PaidaLajin*.

Illness and Healing Reactions are Warnings

Diseases and healing reactions are natural and positive warnings, telling us our agonies are caused by improper thoughts and behaviors that need to be changed, or our condition will worsen. Both arise to maintain our wellbeing.

The only difference between the two is diseases are manifestations of hidden health problems, and healing reactions occur when a person uncovers and resolves the problems. They are two sides of the same coin.

Illness and healing reactions are uncomfortable. People who don't understand their function may be afraid of, hate, or curse them. Please note, each reaction serves a purpose.

Pain

Wherever there is pain, there is a health problem. Taking painkillers only covers up the problem—it does not address the root causes.

Fever

A fever is the body's instinctive reaction when expelling cold. Forcing down a fever by taking medicine may temporarily suppress the symptoms, but seeds of future diseases are planted. It takes away the immune system's ability to fight illness.

High Blood Pressure

Meridian blockages and high blood viscosity hinder *qi* and blood circulation. The heart instinctively increases the pressure to enable the blood to push through the blockages.

If the root causes of diseases are not pinpointed for targeted treatment, and drugs are blindly taken to suppress symptoms, not only will the diseases not be cured: more problems will arise later on. People who have taken long-term medication have experienced this.

Now that we know diseases and healing reactions are signs of our self-healing instinct to love, protect, and heal the body, we should be grateful for them and not disregard or misinterpret the messages. By experiencing healing reactions, we have the opportunity to discover root causes—and correct them.

Healing Reactions Test Your Mind

Healing reactions are recovery responses. Whether they are regarded as something good or bad depends on a person's mindset. If you are negative, worried, fearful, and prone to complaining, diseases will be perceived as deadly risks. If you are positive, reflective, grateful, and willing to change yourself, diseases will be perceived as helpful warnings. Illness and healing test our bodies, but even more so, they test our minds. This can be a turning point in your life.

Diseases originate in the Heart and are cured by heartfelt changes. When discomfort is viewed with negativity and fear, they are perceived as diseases. When viewed with gratitude, they begin the healing process.

If you suffer from weak *qi* and blood flow, and the reactions are severe, take some time to rest, drink ginger and jujube tea, and reduce the intensity of *PaidaLajin*. You can spread out the time you do the practice as well, to match your comfort level.

After your condition improves, continue *PaidaLajin*. People with weak *qi* and blood, the seriously ill, and people who are elderly or frail need more *PaidaLajin*. Slap gently, but don't stop. When the meridians are blocked, it is hard for the body to absorb nutrients. That's why smoothly flowing meridians are the best nourishment. You will absorb your food better when your *qi* improves.

PaidaLajin exercises should be adopted as life-long habits. In our daily lives, we will still experience damaging thoughts and actions. Practicing *PaidaLajin* daily is similar to eating regular meals. It enables the body to produce, *in vivo*, the best organic nutrition and medicine. *PaidaLajin* can be discontinued during the time you don't experience any side effects, no matter how intensely you do the exercises. This indicates bones are in place and tendons are flexible. However, even yoga teachers with very flexible tendons generally experience signs of detoxification after thirty minutes.

Taoism and The Stages of a Healing Crisis

Healing reactions can occur when you practice *yoga, t'ai chi, qi gong*, meditation, and other traditional exercises. Taoism clearly interprets the phenomena.

Generally, a healing reaction goes through the following three stages:

1. Identifying the Location of Blockages

When *qi* flow is hindered by greater resistance from blockages in the body and can't go through a problem area, it will find an alternative route. Such a process will repeatedly kick in when *qi* encounters other blockages at the alternative routes. These continuous attempts can help remove minor problems, while revealing more severe ones the body can't address yet.

2. Revealing Illness

Persistent practice enhances the *yang* energy. The stronger energy will focus on the identified blockages and charge at them with greater force. As a result, various symptoms will worsen, followed by the revelation of all sorts of illness.

This is when the body is embattled; it is experiencing the most critical stage. Symptoms will be aggravated. Medical check-ups at that time will most likely indicate abnormalities. That is why this stage is dubbed the *dà sǐ dà huó* (大死大活, death and revival) stage. It is the darkness before dawn breaks. Unfortunately, many fail to understand and stop their practice halfway through. Without this dire state of suffering, it is impossible to achieve a body overhaul—and the resulting new lease on life.

3. Fighting Illness

After *qi*'s repeated attempts to go through the problem areas, the body's energy is boosted by continued efforts. Under the constant pressure of increased *qi* flow, the problems will gradually recede and eventually disappear. You will feel the symptoms subsiding—and eventually going away entirely.

The more I study and practice *PaidaLajin*, the more I am amazed by the unfathomable design of human beings. It's totally beyond human comprehension and imagination. The function is so complicated, and yet it's so user friendly. We can see and feel that the human body could only be designed by superior wisdom—and with extreme love. It cannot be an accidental combination of different elements. It's a miracle. We can conclude that self-healing is just like the air we breathe and the sunshine we enjoy daily: they are all free miracles created by the Universe. We don't have to know the details to enjoy them. We just need to have faith.

3

THE MOST IMPORTANT ORGANS IN CHINESE MEDICINE

The heart is the most important organ.

Every Chinese person knows the saying, "Illnesses originate from the Heart."

However, not everyone understands the meaning.

The Chinese character for illness 病 (*pinyin*: *bìng*) has two components: 疒 (health problem) and 丙 (*pinyin*: *bǐng*), which corresponds to Heart fire. Ancient Chinese people believed all diseases come from the Heart. Otherwise they are not 病 (illnesses), but 疾 (*pinyin*: *jí*) with two components 疒 (health problem) and 矢 (*pinyin*: *shǐ*), which literally means "arrows"—external, damaging forces.

When our Heart is weak, stressed out, or contaminated, we get sick or act ignorantly. Since illnesses originate from the Heart—it's the first organ to become sick. The word refers to both the physical organ and the invisible Heart that determines how we feel and lead our lives. All diseases are, in essence, different manifestations of chaos in the invisible Heart. On the physical level, all illnesses are Heart diseases.

The kidneys are the second most important organ.

All Chinese men know the significance of renal function. However, they don't feel they can control it. The kidney energy continually depletes from a person's birth to death. Weakening of renal function in women leads to insomnia, headaches, constipation, hair loss, waist pain, knee pain, menstrual pain, irregular periods, or frequent urination. With enough kidney energy, a person's bones are strong and their brain works well; otherwise the person will suffer from bone loss and forgetfulness. People with deficient kidney energy will feel weak, pained, and cold around their waists. Wall hitting is often a good self-healing choice for deficient kidney energy.

The liver is the third most vital organ.

If you observe the Liver Meridian in a meridians chart, you will find it circles around the genital organs internally and externally. And ancient Chinese dubbed the penis *zong jin* (the reproductive tendon.) According to Chinese Medicine, the liver governs the tendons. Hence, the liver is the governor of the penis.

The urinary bladder is the fourth most significant organ.

Urine and sperm share the same passage in the penis. As the kidneys and urinary bladder are paired to govern the water channels in the body, they thrive and wither together. The health of the prostate, which impacts the health of the penis, is directly influenced by the Urinary Bladder Meridian. Most men over sixty have prostate disorders, whose main symptoms are urgent, frequent, and incomplete urination. They go to the bathroom many times at night.

Prostate disorders impact sleep and sexual function. The urinary bladder is also the largest detoxification channel in the body, so the health of the Urinary Bladder Meridian impacts the liver, spleen, and kidneys. Edema results from blockages in the Kidney and Urinary Bladder Meridians.

I have used acupuncture, acupressure, bone setting, and other external therapies to successfully unblock meridian blockages. However, only a handful of people can afford these therapies.

Stretching on a *Lajin* bench is much cheaper and perhaps even more effective. During *Lajin*, the meridians closely linked to sexual function are dredged to varying degrees. All tendons and ligaments, and almost all of the main meridians in the body are being stretched at one time.

It is an open secret among the men who persist in *PaidaLajin* practice that it greatly boosts their sexual function. An obvious sign is the restored morning erection in many middle-aged and older men. During one *PaidaLajin* seminar, a chiropractor from Los Angeles said sexual functioning is at the top of the *Lajin* benefits list in both men and women.

In addition to *PaidaLajin*, waist swirling, *tie qiang gong*, and wall hitting are simple and effective exercises for quickly boosting sexual functioning. You can find directions for these in the *Other Qi Exercises and Meditation* section of this book.

Although I'm talking about sexual function from the perspective of a man, these exercises are applicable to women as well. The meridians in men and women are located in the same places. The impact of *qi* on a man's penis is the same as its impact on a woman's breasts and genitals. In a word, sufficient *qi* makes things full, while deficient *qi* results in apathy and atrophy.

Breasts play a significant role in a woman's sex life. However, they can become a warehouse of toxins and wastes.

Nine meridians pass through or near the breasts: the Ren, Heart, Pericardium, Lung, Liver, Spleen, Kidney, Stomach, and Gall Bladder Meridians. When these meridians are clogged, a woman will suffer from a lot of diseases, including depression, heart disease, uterine fibroids, thyroid disorders, and breast tumors. A female fitness expert wrote that all breast-beautifying therapies, whether physical, chemical, surgical, or implants, have side effects. *PaidaLajin* is the most natural and healthy way to improve the appearance of a woman's breasts, because there are no unpleasant or unhealthy side effects.

If you have sexual dysfunction, you can practice *PaidaLajin* to self-heal. If you do not have sexual disorders, you can still practice *PaidaLajin* to enhance your sexual function and create a healthy, sexy glow. Your stamina and physique will improve.

However, if your only or primary motivation for practicing *PaidaLajin* is increasing or restoring your libido: remember sexual satisfaction is not equal to happiness. But health management opens the door to life management and greater happiness.

4

ADDRESSING THREE TYPES OF ILLNESS WITH *PAIDALAJIN*

The *qi* flow follows a law of its own, regardless of a person's will or perception. It reveals both known and unknown illness. This may cause confusion and anxiety. Some think their practice has gone wrong—the existing illness is still there, and new diseases are being produced by the practice. In actual fact, these are natural, desired effects. You can't just resolve the existing problems, you need to have the body go through a thorough, comprehensive healing process. Only then can such a process be considered a complete overhaul of the body.

PaidaLajin targets the following:

1. **Past Injuries and Illnesses**
   Some may have been cured years ago. However, during the healing process, tissues undergo changes, often related to tissue adhesion and scars. Meridian blockages may have existed in these areas. *Qi* at these locations would cause pain in an apparent relapse, but they are simply healing—once and for all.

2. **Existing Illnesses**
   This type refers to existing sicknesses you're aware of. When *qi* hits at the problem areas, you may suffer more severe symptoms.

3. **Future Illnesses**
   Future illnesses fall into three sub-categories:

- Existing illnesses with a current lack of obvious symptoms
- Illnesses that doesn't show symptoms in early stages, such as deficient kidney energy, stagnating liver energy, or excessive heart fire
- Latent illnesses that will manifest in the future, if you don't address your health

You will feel their presence when healing occurs, even if they haven't been diagnosed yet.

Persistence is essential for those who want to self-heal. Experiencing healing reactions is an important and necessary step toward recovery. Only when you go through this stage, can you heal from all past, existing, and latent health problems—and be assured of future good health.

5

HOW DOES *PAIDALAJIN* WORK?

"Pain Medicine" is Nourishing

Smoothly flowing meridians are the best nourishment. Thus, 'pain medicine' is good nourishment.

Removing the excess and replenishing the deficiency is a principle of health management advocated in Chinese Medicine. Some people assume *PaidaLajin* removes the excess but does not replenish the deficiency. They fear doing *PaidaLajin* for an extended period might reduce their already low energy. This is a misconception.

The magic of *PaidaLajin* is it brings about both effects.

When it comes to replenishing the deficiency, many people think about eating. Chinese people have infinite reasons to eat. They especially love nourishing foods and supplements. When people get sick, their first thought is to eat something nutritious. Gifts are often in the form of various foods and supplements. But are they nourishing the body or growing diseases? In fact, many conditions are created by excessive eating, drinking, or supplementation.

Here is a great secret: When the meridians in the body are blocked, excessive consumption does not nourish the body. It cultivates the following conditions:

- Unhealthy weight gain
- Lumps
- Phlegm
- Tumors
- Inflammation
- Cold-dampness

These abnormalities need nutrition to grow. Like the wild grass in a rice field, they are better at grabbing nutrition than normal cells. They can grow faster when a patient blindly takes supplements. By clearing meridians, you replenish the deficiency by allowing your body to properly absorb nutrition from normal sources—without the need for supplementation.

Here's a real-life example:

A woman almost self-healed her uterine fibroids by practicing *PaidaLajin*, but then she was advised to take supplements. She spent a lot of money on sheep placenta injections. The uterine fibroids grew again.

As we all know, all medication is more or less toxic. Avoid medication unless absolutely necessary. Vitamins, calcium tablets, and other supplements are no exception. They are not benign and taking too much can cause many health problems. The many recalls of drugs and supplements are telling.

Nourishing the Body

When the roads, gas, water, and power lines in a city are blocked, do we solve the problem by increasing vehicles, gas, water, and electricity? Of course not.

The pressing task is to clear the roads and dredge the pipelines. Similarly, we must unclog meridians. Nutrients can't work their way through the blockages, so abnormal growth occurs at them. When they grab nutrition there it grows wildly; diseases will proliferate. *PaidaLajin* methodically disintegrates these abnormalities, regulates *qi* and blood circulation, and redistributes nutrition. Your body will automatically remove the excess and replenish the deficiency.

Reducing food intake and fasting enhances your health by removing toxins and abnormal growths in your body, so nutrients and *yang* energy move where they're needed. Imagine if the oil tube linked to the engine is blocked. Can you add more gasoline to make the car run faster? No!

More importantly, *PaidaLajin* also enhances *qi*, which disintegrates the toxins and alien life forms, transforming them. Waste becomes nutrition, and thus enemies become friends.

PaidaLajin kills several birds with one stone. It:

- Detoxifies
- Boosts energy levels
- Reduces excess fat

Treating Diseases and Treating Fate

PaidaLajin is demonstratively effective in relieving or curing acute and chronic joint pain, especially in the shoulders, lower back, buttocks, knees, and legs. But what about chronic diseases? Can *PaidaLajin* self-heal a hundred diseases, including cancer?

The answer is yes.

Here, the numbers indicate the wide scope of *PaidaLajin*'s applicability. No therapy in the world carries the promise of healing everyone. *PaidaLajin* can't cure those who don't believe in it or practice it diligently.

Therapists often say, "We treat diseases, but not fate." If you disbelieve *PaidaLajin* or practice it only when you're terminally ill, isn't it your fate to be sick? You see, the Chinese character "命" (*ming*) means both life and fate.

Those who conscientiously practice *PaidaLajin* have already changed their minds. Confidence, determination, patience, doubt, fear, and contradiction all reflect changes in the mind. The efficacies of *PaidaLajin* vary from one to another, as people have different states of mind. Fluctuations in one's health condition, *PaidaLajin* session length and intensity, and other factors are all related to the mind.

Why is sickness often accompanied by bad luck, while recovery from illness seems to bring good luck? This law of life is well worth contemplating.

For much of human history, humanity did not depend on the medical community. Thanks to the ability to self-heal, we have survived until today. Self-healing follows natural laws. Chinese people summarized the natural law and named it The *Tao* (The Way.) They believe The *Tao* is the source of everything in the universe, and it appears in different ways. Self-healing and the human body are products of creation 造化 (or however you prefer to name the universal life force.)

It has two connotations: 造 (to create) and 化 (to change; to transport and to transform.) In other words, humans are a product of prenatal and postnatal influences. For us, the initial creation is a bygone past. However, we can actively transform our lives at the present time.

How can such simple exercises create healing miracles?

There are clear scientific interpretations and very encouraging clinical research results included later in the book. And we welcome other researchers and medical institutions to conduct independent research into *PaidaLajin*.

We analyzed years of clinical results and thousands of testimonials. We drew inspiration from relevant theories of Classical Chinese Medicine (CCM) and cutting-edge modern science. Here are some interpretations for your reference:

PaidaLajin from the Perspective of Chinese Medicine

When *yang* energy rises, *yin* energy falls, and vice versa. The *yin* and *yang* energies constantly re-organize until they eventually reach equilibrium. A healthy person is well balanced. Getting sick indicates a *yin-yang* imbalance, which is invariably caused by meridian blockages.

All Chinese therapies, including cupping, bone setting, skin scraping, acupuncture, acupressure, moxibustion, and herbal medicine are aimed at clearing meridian blockages. The same is true with *PaidaLajin*—only it works more efficiently.

The overall trend of a person's health from birth to death is rising *yin* energy and declining *yang* energy. *PaidaLajin* boosts *yang* energy and curbs *yin* energy. During this process, pain and diseases are naturally self-healed—and it has a proven anti-aging effect.

There are many natural, holistic therapies. Each is precious in its own way. Due to various reasons, it is a challenge to share most of these therapies on a large scale. *PaidaLajin* has great overall healing effects for everyone, and it is complementary to other therapies.

Differences between *PaidaLajin* and other TCM therapies

PaidaLajin is a self-healing exercise ordinary people can practice on their own or with others. Its core feature is voluntary practice; other Traditional Chinese Medicine (TCM) therapies are normally dependent upon professionals.

According to Chinese Medicine, the Heart is the King of Bodily Organs and its power is the greatest. When a person voluntarily practices *PaidaLajin*, the power of the Heart is fully mobilized. This initiates a fundamental change in the nature of healing. By contrast, when a person receives medication and other interventions, much of this power is wasted. It can even lead to more problems than it solves.

PaidaLajin's scope, depth, and intensity go far beyond other therapies. If you have doubts about this claim, join a workshop and experience it for yourself. It can also be proven in generally-accepted scientific experiments.

PaidaLajin from the Perspectives of Science and Western Medicine

From this perspective, there are infinite mysteries in *PaidaLajin*, waiting to be unraveled.

To establish scientific evidence:

- Use universally acknowledged research methods
- Properly observe subjects
- Reliably record data
- Ensure results are repeatable

PaidaLajin meets all these research requirements.

Now, let us put aside hypotheses. We will compare Western and Chinese Medicine to explain how *PaidaLajin* works and use Western Medicine explanations for clarity.

CHINESE MEDICINE	WESTERN MEDICINE
Holistic	Based on Specific Parts
Balance the Body	Treat the Symptoms
Invisible Systems	Visible Systems

PaidaLajin Produces Vibrations

Everything in the universe vibrates, be it visible or invisible, audible or inaudible. *PaidaLajin* produces rhythmic vibrations, just like percussion and orchestral music. It changes the vibration patterns and frequencies of all organs and cells and produces resonance in the body. This helps to normalize discordant frequencies of cells, atoms, electrons, and molecules in the body. It is like tuning noisy instruments to create beautiful melodies. We can regain health by getting rid of the noises (pathogenic elements) in the body.

PaidaLajin changes the frequency of the heart. Consequently, the vibration patterns and frequencies of all other organs and cells are changed. Perhaps unbeknownst to many people, all organs and cells have their respective vibration patterns and frequencies. They are like invisible rainbows and inaudible music to us, due to our limited sensory functions. A healthy body resembles a symphony, and an unhealthy body is a chaotic mess. The human heart is the conductor of this live-performance symphony orchestra.

A person becomes sick when the frequency of a part of the body (a musical instrument) becomes discordant with the overall frequency (the entire band.) Chinese Medicine explains it as the generating-inhibiting interactions of the Five Elements (wood, fire, earth, metal, and water) in the body. In other words, organs with different attributes vibrate at different frequencies and interact with each other to create what are called interference waves in physics.

A constructive interference is a generating interaction among organs; a destructive interference is an inhibiting interaction among organs. Chinese Medicine advocates the treatment philosophy of maintaining good balance—removing the excess and replenishing the deficiency.

Western Medicine is focused on tangible systems, such as the nervous and circulatory systems. Chinese Medicine is more concerned with the intangible systems of Essence, *qi*, and Spirit, particularly the invisible *qi*. *Yin* and *yang* energies have different frequencies. Dynamic *yin-yang* equilibrium marks the process of becoming ill and being healed. And *ling shu* (pivot of the soul) refers to the meridians through which *qi* flows.

Western Medicine emphasizes the chemical composition of a drug. Chinese herbal medicine underlines the generating-inhibiting impact of its frequency on *qi*, problem areas, and related meridians. It clears discordant frequencies and eventually makes the body's overall frequency balanced and harmonious, thus healing diseases.

The traditional Chinese character 藥 (medicine) is composed of 艹 (grass, herbs) and 樂 (music)—music grown from herbs or from Heaven.

We can't split a piece of Mozart's music into individual musical notes and attempt to find out which one makes the music great.

Similarly, we can't treat a malfunctioning organ separately, and expect it to be healed regardless of the patient's overall health. Healing is only meaningful when the malfunctioning organ vibrates in sync with the entire system. All Chinese therapies sort out the chaotic mess and create a new balance.

It is easy to apply this theory to *Paida*, because slapping is quite rhythmic. But many people do not understand how *Lajin* produces vibrations or that the more intense *Lajin* is, the higher its frequency is. *Paida* produces percussion music, while *Lajin* makes string music—the yelling, moaning, and breathing during *PaidaLajin* is music played with wind instruments.

In the language of physics, *PaidaLajin* creates both constructive and destructive interference waves. The overall effect is constructive. The interference waves produce pain. The Heart feels pain in every part of the body. It mobilizes all the body's might to instantly improve the condition of damaged regions.

The self-healing power in us knows what to destroy and remove, and what to protect and nourish. This is called "no destruction, no construction". Human life, nature, and the entire universe follow this natural law. *PaidaLajin*'s process of diagnosis and treatment is much safer and more accurate than medical interventions.

6

SELF-HELP *PAIDA*

SELF-HELP *PAIDA*

1. *Paida* involves confidence, concentration, and perseverance.
2. When you believe in self-healing principles, you remain focused and persistent. When effected by negativity, you can't continue with your full attention. The effect will be discounted—even if you continue the practice.
3. Close your eyes and remain silent.
   It is easier to clear your thoughts and focus when your eyes are closed. It also helps you avoid being distracted by what you see, and it makes you less likely to chat with other people.

Understand the Philosophy of Self-Healing Methods

Re-read the previous sections to deepen your understanding, especially concerning healing reactions.

It will boost your confidence in self-healing, and you can read countless testimonials. Millions of people have self-healed with *PaidaLajin*. Why not you?

Be Grateful

Positive and negative energies do not exist alone. If there is still hatred and resentment in you, the seed of illness is not eliminated. Gratitude is the best way to clear negativity.

1. Be grateful to the Universal Life Force that created everything and to your body, for urging you to change your bad habits.
2. Appreciate your body. If you keep exploiting it, you will continue to be sick.
3. If you're already sick and angry with your body, it is only natural your condition will worsen.
4. Be grateful to your parents and country for nurturing you, and to people—alive or dead—who have helped and cared for you. You can think of their names and faces during the *Paida* process.
5. Express similar gratitude to your enemies and those who have hurt you. Like those who have helped you in positive ways, they are indispensable to your growth as a person.
6. Combine gratitude and repentance together. You can chant aloud or silently, "I'm sorry; please forgive me; thank you; I love you." These powerful phrases are used in the Hawaiian Healing System. You can read more in *Zero Limits: The Secret Hawaiian System for Wealth, Health, Peace, and More*, authored by Joe Vitale and Dr. Ihaleakala Hew Len.

Fill Yourself with Clean *Qi* and Expel Dirty *Qi*

Imagine your body being filled with clean *qi* from the palm of your hand. When you remove your palm, think of dirty *qi* being drawn out and expelled from your body.

Recite Mantras

You can recite a mantra out loud or in your Heart. For instance, Christians may chant "Hallelujah". Buddhists may chant "Amitabha" or "Om Mani Padme Hum."

Pay Attention to Your Breathing

Whether you are slapping or being slapped, you can inhale through your nose, hold your breath for three seconds to a minute—or even longer—and exhale rapidly through your mouth. It helps relieve the pain, boosts *yang*, and rids your body of foul air. You can observe your breathing and sensations calmly and objectively. It helps you become aware of sensations, both pleasant and unpleasant.

7

MUTUAL *PAIDA*

When engaged in mutual slapping, it's important to maintain a caring heart, a positive mindset, and hope for a fast recovery.

Both the slapper and the recipient need to relax physically and psychologically, particularly the area being treated. Psychological relaxation is even more vital, because when you feel nervous, your body will be tense, increasing your pain.

1. Maintain good communication.
2. Pay attention to words, actions, and facial expressions. Both parties should stay focused and connected as 'one'.
3. Do not talk during *Paida*. It consumes energy and it's distracting. Ideally, all you hear is the rhythmic sounds of slapping.
4. Always start with gentle *Paida* before gradually increasing the intensity.
5. The intensity and technique can be adjusted at any time.
6. Make sure the intensity is within everyone's pain tolerance.
7. Never force heavy *Paida* on anyone.
8. Express gratitude to each other.

Fear and resentment in the recipient will reduce the healing effect instead of enhancing it.

Heavy *Paida* is not suitable for infants, the elderly, and the seriously ill. Gentle *Paida* can produce the same healing effect as expected or even better, if you *Paida* long enough—and with love.

Negative Energy During *Paida*

According to Isaac Newton's third law of motion, the intensity of slapping will equal the intensity of being slapped.

So, when you use your hands to slap others, your palms are being slapped as well. Our coaches help participants learn to slap in workshops all year round. They are not damaged by negative energy; instead, they are getting healthier.

Nonetheless, some people will be overly concerned, and they might think themselves into uncomfortable emotions. Also, some people are very susceptible to the impact of external energy.

TIPS:

1. First of all, enhance your personal positive energy.
2. Persistent *PaidaLajin*, meditation, and meditative standing (also called *zhan zhuang* or "Horse Stance") are good ways to boost your energy level.
3. If you are a theist, silently pray to your Creator, God, or Buddha for protection.
4. You can also chant mantras.
5. After mutual *Paida*, swing and shake your hands and feet.
6. It is even better to stand barefoot on the soil or grass.

8

SHA AND SELF-HEALING

***Sha* (痧; *pinyin: shā*)**

Sha is toxic waste in the blood and bodily fluids. It appears beneath the skin during *Paida*.

It can be pink, crimson, purple, purplish black, or black.

When the amount of *sha* reaches a peak, it will gradually fade away with continued *Paida*. Lumps, red swelling, and white powder on the skin are different forms of *sha*.

Sha is a unique word in the Chinese language. It literally means "toxic sands and little stones". Ancient Chinese called them blood stones, pathogenic substances similar to gall bladder stones and kidney stones. Establishing its occurrence and coining the term *sha*, as well as using it to diagnose and treat disease, demonstrates the wisdom of the ancient Chinese people.

In scientific language, *sha* refers to tiny, toxic particles being processed and filtered. When *PaidaLajin* boosts *yang* energy, it induces biochemical reactions with various substances in the body. *Qi* excretes these particles through various orifices, including sweat, tears, nasal discharge, urine, and stool.

Four Types of Toxins in *Sha*

1. Environmental-force toxins like wind, heat, cold, and dampness.
2. Disease-oriented toxins.
3. Toxins from prolonged medication and processed food. You might smell chemical odors during *Paida*.

4. Toxins caused by negative emotions. These are far more toxic than the others. They are the main cause of illness.

Paida forces toxic waste in the blood to cling to blood vessel walls. Colorful patches of *sha* appear beneath the skin. With the same intensity of *Paida*, *sha* does not appear on healthy acupoints.

Self-Diagnosis: Including Color

- *Sha* only appears when you're ill
- The amount of *sha* indicates the severity of each disease
- The darker the *sha*, the more severe the pathogenic elements (such as toxic waste, excessive cold, heat, or dampness)
- Swollen lumps may appear with *sha*
- Regardless of the disease name, after *sha* decomposes, the illness is healed
- *Sha* might not appear where we expect it to
- Heavy *Paida* on a healthy person doesn't create very much *sha*
- Gentle *Paida* on a sick person produces a lot of *sha*

Implications

Flushed Skin: healthy and normal

Red: Wind heat—common in people with poor health

Purplish Red: Stagnant heat—prone to feeling sore

Blue: Phlegm-dampness—prone to fatigue

Purplish Black: Stagnation and inflammation, indicating heavy meridian blockages

Black: Appearing mostly with chronic or critical illnesses, or after prolonged medication

Colorful *Sha* and Swollen Skin: Severe blockages

1. *Sha* indicates detoxification is underway—excessive heat, cold, dampness, and toxic waste in related organs are being expelled.
2. *Sha* appears more rapidly in severely blocked meridians often in under a minute. However, pain is a more accurate way to diagnose a block than *sha*.
3. Some *sha* travels in the body. *Qi* and blood flow are being regulated by *Paida*.
4. *Sha* may be red at first, but darker spots, lines, or patches might appear. In severe cases, even dark, hard lumps emerge.
5. *Sha* may not come out easily in seriously ill people, because *qi* is weak and it fails to stimulate blood circulation. People with insufficient *qi* and blood may have rough skin that's hard to stimulate. If the toxins are buried deeply, it might be harder to get them out. It may take additional work.
6. Sometimes *sha* disappears after a few sessions but re-appears later. When, where, and how much *sha* doesn't match up with a person's willpower. Sometimes, no matter how hard you slap, no *sha* will come out. Other times, it will surface unexpectedly. A person's health condition is constantly changing. In that tug-of-war with *qi*, toxins are changing and moving around all of the time.
7. If *sha* appears only when you receive *Paida* from someone else, you're probably being too gentle with yourself. Increase the intensity of your practice.
8. During illnesses, *sha* will appear in different places, and *Paida* will hurt more.

9. *Sha* might quickly turn lighter, become yellow, or have a pale, wave-like shade. It might spread to surrounding areas. These are all normal reactions, indicating *qi* and blood is traveling to all previously blocked body tissues.

Sha, Qi, and Blood

Sha will appear on the same body in various shades, colors, and patterns. In more severe cases, *sha* may look horrifying. It is normal for *sha* to hurt when touched or rubbed.

The *yin* toxins of *sha* will gradually warm up with *Paida*—rising *yang* energy. Sometimes when you're sick, you feel hot one minute and cold the next. This is *yin* and *yang* energies wrestling inside your body. Cold hands and feet during and after *Paida* show that cold is being expelled.

Sha is a very vivid manifestation of *yin-yang* interactions. Like the bellows that Lao Tse described in the *Tao Te Ching*, when *yang* rises, *yin* subsides. Diseases are healed, and *yin-yang* energies attain balance. Diseases improve as *sha* and swelling fade away. The effect is similar in gua *sha* (skin scraping) and ba guan (cupping) therapies.

Everyone can benefit from *PaidaLajin*.

Elderly people in their 80s or 90s experience very visible improvements after *PaidaLajin*. Gently patting a child under a year old is even more effective than slapping an adult, because an infant has strong *yang* and fully accepts the positive energy without the interference of culture and knowledge.

Children with severe tendon stiffness should start practicing *PaidaLajin* now—rather than later on in life.

9

WHAT IS HEALTHY LIVING?

Imagine we were born just a few months ago. Our bodies are in perfect shape. Our skin is soft and milky. We're constantly smiling and worry-free. We love everyone. We have no enemies, and everyone loves us. In short, we are happy, healthy, and full of energy.

What happened to us?

We're busy. We consume various stimulants. We gradually become disappointed with life, with people, with our job—or perhaps we should say—with the entire world. Our health begins to deteriorate. Our energy begins to lag. We become unhappy and frustrated. And we often procrastinate until we become really sick. Then we see a doctor, take some medicine, or have surgery.

Are you in this kind of situation?

Why wait until your condition becomes alarmingly worse?

Our bodies are complete, self-sustaining systems. The intricacies and subtleties of the human body aren't understood yet. But if we follow natural rhythms, we can stay healthy. To live a happy, healthy, and meaningful life, we need to listen to our inner voice, find out who we really are, and lead a green, balanced lifestyle. It's easier said than done, but it's not only worthwhile—it's necessary.

Huang Di Nei Jing on healthy living

Huang Di Nei Jing, a Chinese medical classic compiled over two millennia ago, provides treasured guidelines to doctors and common-sense knowledge on healthy living. Its wisdom still rings true today.

It's easy to recover when your body gets sick. It's more difficult when your Heart is sick, and even worse when your soul gets sick.

The body, Heart, and soul are connected. When one is hurt, all are hurt. The Heart is the center. It can get sick, but it can also be healed. People who think too much don't have peace in their Heart. They are usually negative, get sick often, and have difficulty recovering. Even when they recover, the Heart easily gets sick again, leading to other illnesses. During *PaidaLajin*, we need to overcome our fear, laziness, and skepticism. These are all illnesses of the Heart that are difficult to heal. This is why the words for fear, laziness, and skepticism in Chinese all have the word Heart embedded in them.

All diseases are connected to the Heart

Disease, or 病 in Chinese, has a component 丙. 丙 means fire according to the Five Elements Theory, which connects to the Heart. Our ancestors explained this through the creation of Chinese characters: All diseases are caused by sickness of the Heart, otherwise they would not be called "diseases" or 病, they would be called 疾. 疾 has a component 矢, which means "arrow" or external damage, and is pronounced with the sound of 急 *ji* (quick, urgent.)

The Heart is hurt the most often and severely, ever since we were little. Children feel hurt when they can't have the candy they want, can't get good grades in school, or when other children's toys or clothes are better than theirs. When they grow up and fall in love, they will almost always experience heartbreak. This is why people say, "My heart is shattered."

Eventually, many of us experience pressure from work, marriage, children, mortgages, and relationships. We overload our hearts to the point we can no longer cope. We become sick from fear, anger, hatred, anxiety, tension, laziness, jealousy, and frustration. These are the opposite of joy, bliss, contentment, and happiness. Negative emotions are similar to being cold. They lead to tightness and contraction of the Heart. This leads to the contraction of all tendons. Eventually, it spreads to our entire bodies.

PaidaLajin heals the Heart through the body. But if we lack confidence, determination, and perseverance, *PaidaLajin* will not work. Even if we recover, we will get sick again.

Self-healing has nothing to do with money

I received a referral from a friend who had convulsions, neck pain, shoulder pain, and chest pain. He had seen many renowned doctors of many disciplines—Western doctors, Chinese doctors, acupuncturists, chiropractors, and others—all in vain. He still suffered from pain and agony.

Me: "You could self-heal with *PaidaLajin*."

Him: "I am really sick. Please help!"

Me: "If you are really sick, then come to a *PaidaLajin* workshop as soon as possible."

Him: "I want to fly you over to America to cure me. I will buy your air ticket and pay for your hotel and your fees."

Me: "I am not a doctor. I do not treat patients. I only run workshops to teach people how to self-heal. Why don't you fly over to the workshop?"

Him: "I am too busy at work."

This is very typical. Many people think they can pay to have their pain and diseases cured. But self-healing is really a wake-up call from within. It has nothing to do with money—but everything to do with the Heart. This guy was so sick, but he still couldn't let go. 忙 (Busy-ness) is made up of the "Heart" and "death" components. So busy-ness means the Heart is dead—or at least numb. Chinese doctors see the Heart not only as a physical organ, but also as energy—a system that can't be seen. Our ancestors called it light from above. Our Heart is our light, our guardian.

The Heart feels agony, pressure, and negative emotions. But doctors, MRIs, electrocardiograms, and other machines can't always detect it. It is easy to believe good test results mean the heart is well. But the Heart unconditionally bears more strain.

People who die young all share one thing: they push their hearts to the extreme before they die.

With this gentleman, it did not matter that I explained to him, "I am not a doctor. I do not cure people. I just teach people to heal themselves." He still wanted me to cure him.

His logic was that his business was very important, and his illness came at a bad time. Treating illness is a doctor's business, so he paid doctors to treat him. When it failed, and he heard *PaidaLajin* would work for him, he wanted to pay money for people to do it for him. I advised him to read my book and blog. After much persuasion, he finally agreed.

The next day, he said, "I read your blog. I am convinced I need *Paida*. Would you please find someone for me? Please!"

I replied, "You can *Paida* your universal regions and stretch on a *Lajin* bench.

He said, "I want to have someone do *Paida* for me. I have no energy to do it myself."

I told him, "Use a *Paida* stick. It saves a lot of energy. You can do *Lajin* on your own."

He asked, "Where should I *Paida*?"

This is a question many people ask. They are reluctant to understand the principles; they just want to heal in a few minutes. This is the logic of medicine: apply treatment to symptoms. Stomachaches can be treated by slapping the *Zusanli* Acupoints, but it's only temporary. Your body is a connected system, and you need to treat it as such.

Diseases are not cured, but healed

Unfortunately, our feelings toward illness are negative. We are filled with hatred.

If we can't love ourselves and simply wait for others to treat us, we won't heal. Diseases are opportunists: whether we let them take hold or not is up to us. Being overly dependent on others amputates our power. You activate your power; others can only assist you.

Money

Some people stop *PaidaLajin* as soon as they recover and jump back into moneymaking and career-ladder climbing. Many are worried about healthcare costs later in life. In this case, their wish will come true—all their hard-earned money goes to the hospital.

If we do not know how to reflect, draw on our own resources, and always view illnesses as an external matter, we won't change. "Remorse" in Chinese is 忏悔. We must ask our bodies for forgiveness. In addition, we need to be genuinely sorry to those we have hurt with our words, actions, and thoughts.

感恩 (grateful) advocates communicating with our hearts and expressing gratitude to our bodies, the universe, and our parents, family, and friends. We must extend it to all beings, people, and things that have helped us grow. We need to feel grateful for *PaidaLajin.*

The best way to express gratitude is to introduce it to more people. Sharing your experience, and encouraging others to self-heal, is definitely no small act. A whole family could be saved because of your testimonial.

The relationship between money and disease

Many diseases are related to money.

If you do not believe me, run a mental evaluation of yourself. Think about how money has impacted you. Money is so mesmerizing. This is why Jesus said, "For where your treasure is, there your heart will be also." The key point isn't how much money you have, but your attitude toward money—which relates to your Heart. Many countries are experiencing great difficulties in medical reform. This is because they are on the wrong money path.

As the saying goes, "There are no small acts of evil." Accumulated small acts of evil will lead to catastrophes. Disease is one example of catastrophe. There is a reason for all disease. Money is intertwined with disease, bad luck, good luck, and longevity. The fate of individuals, countries, and all of humanity is made by us during these action-reaction cycles.

The relationship between image and disease

Why is it some people are prosperous in their careers, and have a happy family and successful children—yet suddenly die young? The answer is simple: pretense.

Many people do not live their lives honestly. They protect their image, while suffering inside. People who pretend to have a perfect life are often the most miserable. Lots of clinical data points to the same conclusion—they suffer from depression, gynecological disorders, and cancer.

If we were to lift the layers of vanity, pretense, illusions, and disease names, we would see the Heart is sick because of attitudes towards money.

Often image and money are interrelated. Many people love brand-name goods for this reason—even if the products aren't superior.

When it comes to *Paida*, some individuals might fear criticism about being unscientific. Being overly concerned with one's looks might make people avoid *sha*. If you care about your looks more than your health and morals, and you only want to be pampered, you will become sick. "Nothing slips through God's net, no matter how sparse the net is."

10

GENERAL ADVICE

Avoid Wind and Chills During *Paida*

Avoid direct wind from an electric fan or an air conditioner during *Paida*. Letting wind and chills enter your body through your pores can induce new illnesses. If air conditioning has to be used, turn the fan to low, and increase the temperature to no less than 79°F (26℃.)

The Best Way to Drink Water with *Paida*

Before, during, and after *Paida*, drink some warm water to replenish fluids, prevent fatigue and dizziness, and enhance your metabolism. Ginger and jujube tea is even better, particularly for those with weak *qi* and blood.

Many people drink water as a habit, even when they are not thirsty. Some even drink gallons a day, which can cause illness. According to Chinese Medicine: drink only when you are thirsty—and drink it warm. Do not assume that drinking water helps detoxification. Where there are blockages, excess water can't help with detoxification. It can get trapped, damaging kidney and urinary bladder functions, and causing other issues.

Cold water, especially in the early morning when *yang* energy rises along with the sun, extinguishes the Heart fire and leads to heart disease.

Avoid Bathing or Showering After *Paida*

1. In cold weather, when you sweat less, don't bathe on the day you do *Paida*.

2. *Qi* and blood flow is automatically enhanced by *PaidaLajin*; don't interfere with this process. Cold-dampness can easily enter the pores when they're wide open from the warm water.
3. On warmer days, shower two hours after *Paida*.
4. Never shower in cold water.
5. Avoid shampoo and shower gels. They contain harmful chemicals.

Continue Until *Sha* Disappears

- This process can take a long time—sometimes over an hour.
- Prolonged *Paida* helps the *sha* fade away faster.
- The slapped area gathers more *qi* and blood, facilitating flow and detoxification.
- On its own, *sha* will disappear in a few hours or days, but it sometimes takes longer.
- If *sha* disappears quickly, it is indicative of good health.
- Normally, *sha* on young, healthy people disappears faster.
- It goes away more slowly in elderly people and gravely ill patients. Severe *sha* might not disappear for weeks.
- After *sha* appears, you can move on to other body parts; wait until *sha* disappears to start a second round on the same area.

***Sha* Isn't Broken Blood Vessels**

Rather, the toxic substances in the blood are decomposing and being removed through pores, other orifices, and detoxification channels in the body.

Sweat, tears, a runny nose, urine, stool, smells from the skin, and other excretions are all telling signs of detoxification.

Dark reddish *sha* that manifests with swollen skin can look horrible. Some people can't put on their shoes after *Paida*, due to swelling. In these cases, continue *Paida*. Don't panic, even if your skin breaks and blood seeps out. *Paida* for a while to get rid of toxic blood and bodily fluids. Then move on to an adjacent area.

Sha and Bleeding Are Part of the Self-Healing Process

When checked with medical equipment, the major blood vessels around the area remain intact. If you slap healthy parts of your body, no *sha* or blood comes out.

It is Normal for Your Skin to Break

You can stop slapping it and move to another region. However, to heal certain illnesses, it is better to *Paida* until the skin breaks, allowing toxic blood and fluids to drain. For instance, people with psoriasis or eczema can get rid of more toxins at the damaged areas. To relieve severe heart disease, slap on the inner elbows until the skin breaks.

CAUTION:

Paida is prohibited in these cases:

1. Those who tend to bleed easily or those with blood disorders, such as hemophilia or Henoch-Schonlein Purpura (HSP) or on people with skin trauma or infected skin.
2. If you're bleeding.
3. If you're suffering from acute injuries, severe infections, or fresh bone fractures.

It's all right to slap on regions with muscle and soft tissue damage and surrounding areas, although the pain will be greater.

CAUTION:

Avoid *Paida* around your eyes if you have detaching retinas.

Duration and Frequency of *PaidaLajin* Practice

1. Whether you're sick or healthy, and whether you see *sha* or not, it's best to practice *PaidaLajin* every day.
2. A long, continuous session of *PaidaLajin* is better than several short sessions.
3. When you have enough time, it's best to thoroughly slap a region for up to thirty minutes. If you don't have that much time, *Paida* one or two regions a day. Thorough *Paida* involves slapping until *sha* appears and continues until it fades away or totally disappears.
4. You can practice *PaidaLajin* anytime and anywhere, conditions permitting.

11

LAJIN PRINCIPLES

Lajin **(拉筋; *pinyin: lā jīn*): *la*, to stretch; *jin*, tendons and ligaments.**

To put it simply, *Lajin* is simple and effective exercises to stretch the tendons and ligaments that connect the skeleton and organs.

Lajin:

- Increases tendon flexibility
- Removes meridian blockages
- Enables smooth *qi* and blood flow

Persistent practice heals various contraction-induced diseases, including the obvious pain existing in the neck, shoulders, waist, and legs.

While *Lajin*, compared with medication and acupuncture, is not widely practiced as a major therapy, various stretching exercises have long existed in *yoga*, sports, *Taoism, kungfu*, *qi gong*, and Chinese Medicine.

A baby has strong *yang* energy and a very soft body. As a person ages, their body becomes stiffer, their tendons get shorter, and their *yang* energy declines. In old age, a person suffers scoliosis and thus becomes shorter. When a person is dead, the *yang* is used up, and their body is completely stiff. The same is true with animals and plants. Green branches and leaves are tender, flexible, and exuberant; withered ones are hard, fragile, and lifeless. Flexibility indicates abundant *yang*; stiffness signals weak *yang*.

The importance of flexible *jin* is reflected in these Chinese adages:

"Where the bones are in place and *jin* is flexible, *qi* and blood will flow smoothly."

"Extending *jin* by one inch will prolong a life by ten years."

"A person thrives when *jin* is flexible—and perishes when *jin* contracts."

In order to live a long and healthy life, we should make our tendons softer, longer, and more flexible.

Jin-suo means tendon stiffness and contraction. It may seem like it only impacts bodily movements. In fact, it negatively impacts all internal organs.

Our bones, limbs, and internal organs are linked together by tendons, ligaments, and meridians. The twelve main tendons run alongside the twelve main meridians. *Jin-suo* causes meridian blockages and health problems. And it does not occur in certain parts of the body, but in the entire body—and throughout a person's life. The pain of jin-suo can often be instantly relieved by *Lajin*.

Jin-suo is related to all illnesses; *Lajin* helps to heal them.

Lajin, like *Paida*, can easily diagnose disease. When the two are combined, they function as an even more precise diagnostic tool.

It is commonly believed people should stop stretching when they're in pain to avoid further injury. However, stretching is needed to avoid further tightening of the tendons. *Lajin* removes blockages and alleviates the pain—"no pain, no blockages."

It should be noted that *Lajin* should start slowly and be gradually increased in duration and intensity. It's best to combine it with *Paida*, a good diet, and other natural therapies.

Daily *Lajin* is one of the best ways to physically exercise.

Important

Detecting *Jin-Suo*

If your body experiences one following eight symptoms, you are suffering from *jin-suo*:

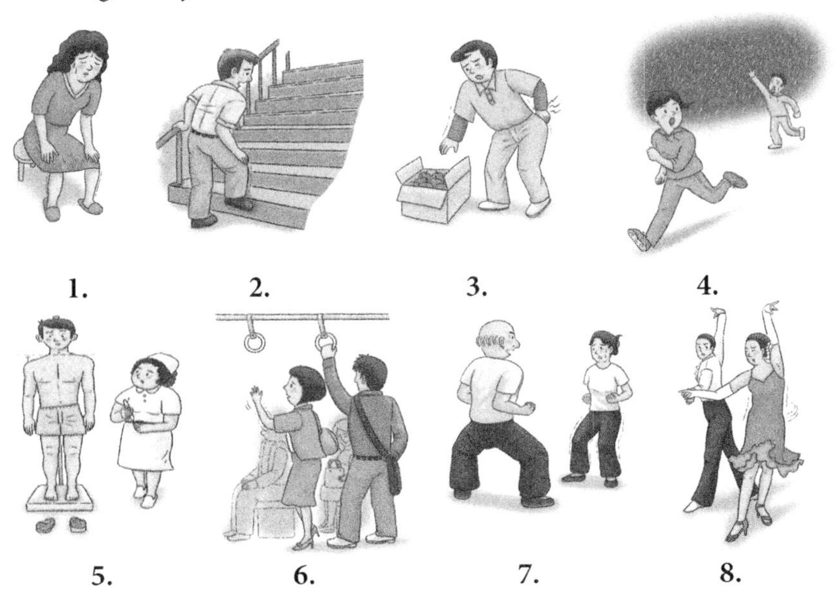

1. **Difficulty Squatting**
   Is it becoming increasingly difficult?
2. **Can You Easily Lift Your Legs?**
   Remember climbing stairs in strides? Is it as easy as it used to be?
3. **Can You Easily Bend at the Waist?**
   Bending becomes increasingly difficult, and you might end up with twists or sprains.
4. **Can You Walk or Run in Long Strides?**
   If you can only take small steps, you are suffering from *jin-suo*.
5. **Is One of Your Legs Longer Than the Other?**
   "How come I never realized it?"
6. **Can You Easily Stretch and Bend Your Arms?**
   Try holding the rings on a bus or train.

7. **Can You Stretch Your Legs from a Seated Position?**
   "Why can't I stretch out as widely as I used to?"
8. **Can You Turn Easily?**
   "Ah, it is not because I am fat—it's because I've got *jin-suo*!"

SIGNS AND SYMPTOMS OF *JIN-SUO*

Flexible *jin* contributes to good health. Once *jin* becomes stiff and shrinks, your body will exhibit one or several of the following symptoms:

- Pain and stiffness in your neck, back, or lumbar region
- Inability to bend down
- Leg pain or paralysis
- Inability to squat
- Uneven legs
- Short steps
- Radiating pain in your heels
- Stressed tendons at your hip joints
- Inability to raise your thighs forward or sideways
- Difficulty turning around
- Contraction of your muscles
- Inability to extend or bend your elbows
- Pain, numbness, swelling, or inflexibility in arms, legs, elbows, or knees
- Diabetes
- Stroke sequelae

Signs of *jin-suo*: When curling your legs, the lowered leg can't touch the ground, and your arms can't rest on the *Lajin* bench.

Jin-suo also contributes to the following problems:

- Excretory Disorders
- Hemorrhoids

- Prostate disorders
- Urinary blockages
- Urgent, frequent, or involuntary urination
- Reproductive disorders
- Menstrual pain
- Irregular menstruation
- Ovarian cysts
- Uterine tumors
- Infertility
- Impotence
- Premature ejaculation
- Seminal emission
- Decreased libido
- Inexplicable internal organ pain
- Stomach pain
- Abdominal pain
- Gastroenteritis
- Children's abdominal pain
- Cold, pain, numbness, and swelling in hands and feet
- Cardiovascular disorders and cerebrovascular diseases
- Hypertension
- Chest tightness
- Shortness of breath
- Irregular heartbeat
- Liver and gall bladder disorders
- Type A Hepatitis
- Type B Hepatitis
- Type C Hepatitis
- Gall bladder inflammation
- Skin diseases
- Psoriasis
- Neurodermatitis
- Allergic dermatitis

THE SEVEN *LAJIN* POSTURES

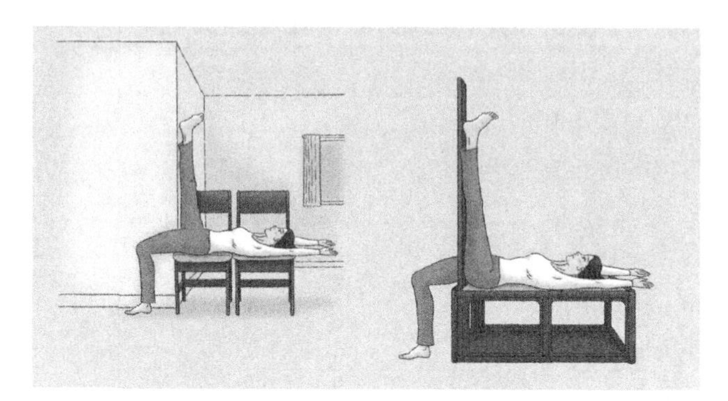

Figure 1: *Lajin* in Reclining Posture

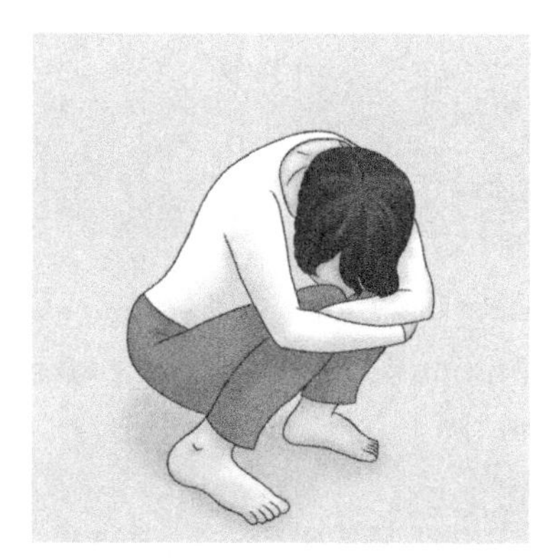

Figure 2: *Lajin* in Squatting Posture

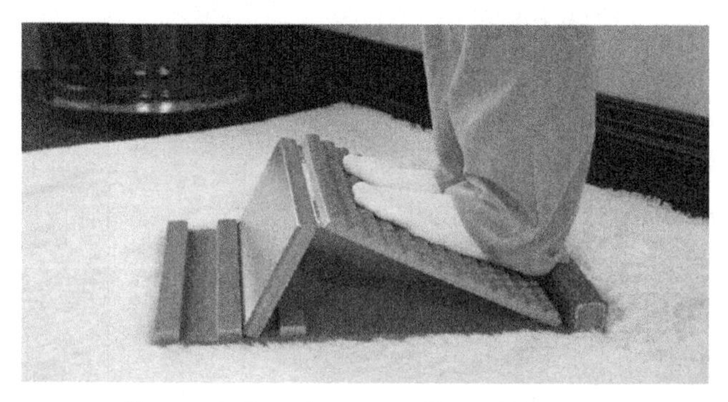

Figure 3: Standing on a Board Posture

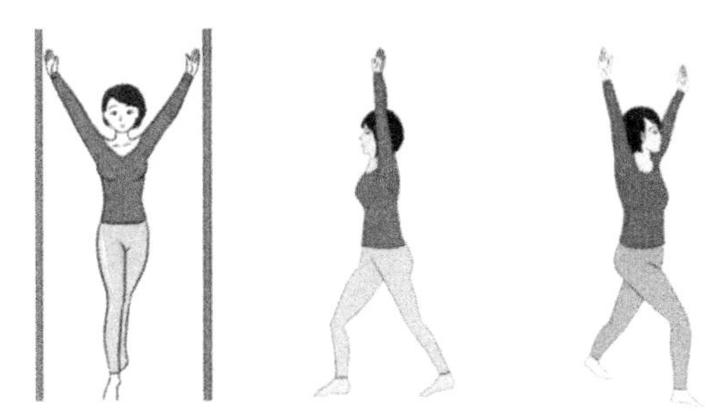

Figure 4: *Lajin* in Standing Posture

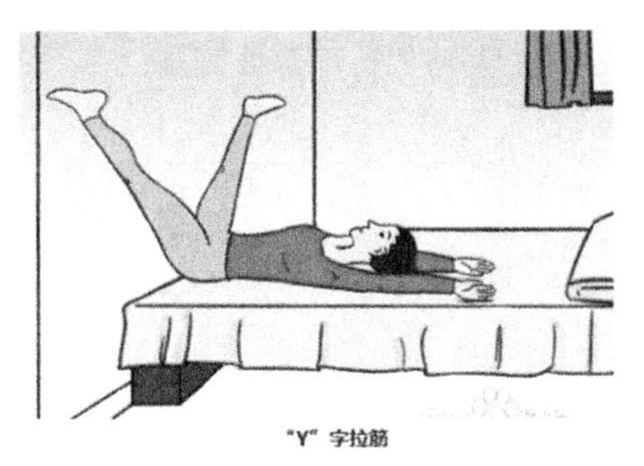

Figure 5: *Lajin* in Y-Shaped Posture

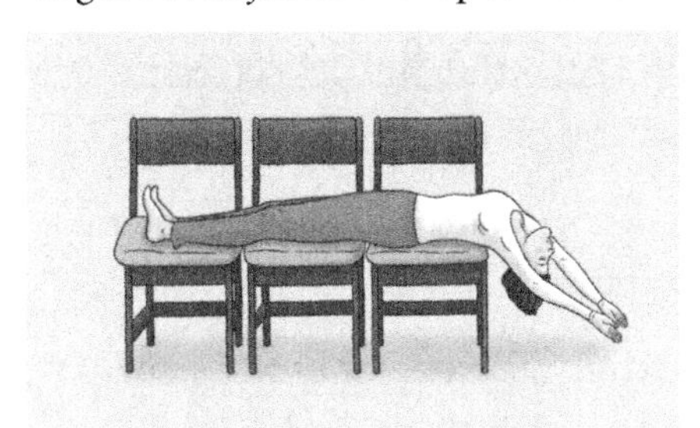

Figure 6: Neck *Lajin*

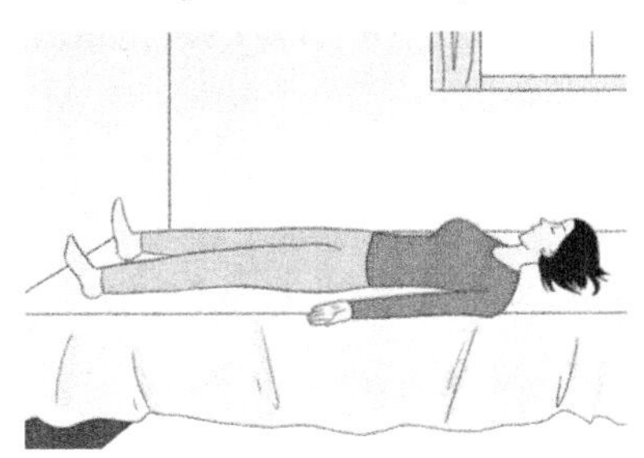

Figure 7: *Lajin* During Sleep

1: RECLINING POSTURE

This is the safest and most useful *Lajin* exercise. It stretches the most tendons and ligaments and dredges all meridians in the body, to varying degrees.

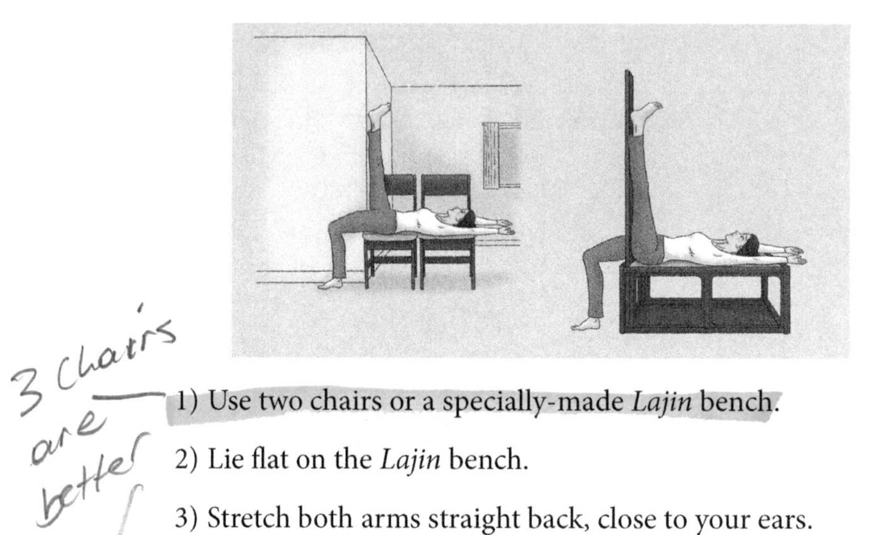

1) Use two chairs or a specially-made *Lajin* bench.
2) Lie flat on the *Lajin* bench.
3) Stretch both arms straight back, close to your ears. They should rest on the bench.
4) Your raised leg should be parallel to the pole with the strap just above your knee.
5) The foot of your raised leg should be at a 90° angle with the pole, turned slightly inward.
6) Your buttocks, the back of your knee, and the heel of your raised leg should press against the pole.
7) Your hip joints, on both sides, should be flat on the bench.
8) The entire sole of your lowered foot should be on the ground.
9) Move your legs closer together.
10) Have someone add sandbags or other weights to your feet and hands to increase the intensity.
11) Stay in this stretch for ten to forty minutes, then switch legs.

If you feel soreness, numbness, pain, or swelling, *Lajin* is working. You can judge the degree of discomfort in someone else by their facial expressions. The more pain, the more healing—but it needs to be kept within the person's pain tolerance.

A beginner may not be able to stretch in a standard way, due to tendon stiffness and contraction. This is normal. Do it daily and gradually increase the time and intensity.

In the absence of a *Lajin* bench, use chairs to stretch by a wall or a doorframe. However, it is only a temporary substitute.

The disadvantages of using chairs:

- They aren't as safe, even, and comfortable
- You can't strap your raised leg to the wall or door frame
- The height of the chairs might vary

You might gain some benefits using chairs, but the *Lajin* bench will significantly increase your healing.

Benefits of Reclining Posture

All meridians are directly or indirectly dredged, particularly the Heart, Pericardium, Liver, Spleen, Kidney, Gall Bladder, and Urinary Bladder Meridians.

This helps to detoxify, heal diseases, and improve immune and sexual functions.

Pain is instantly relieved in the head, neck, back, waist, hips, legs, knees, feet, liver, stomach, gall bladder, and pelvis.

Reclining Posture significantly improves diabetes, hypertension, heart disease, prostatitis (inflammation of the prostate gland), skin, liver, kidney, and stomach diseases, hemorrhoids, constipation, stroke sequelae, and many other conditions.

Its by-products include:

- Increases in height and beauty
- Weight loss
- Fading freckles, wrinkles, and acne

The most striking improvement is seen in the elderly, as many suffer from shrunken tendons.

According to some beauty salon owners, *Lajin* in Reclining Posture, combined with proper breathing, tightens sagging breasts.

In addition to healing lower back and leg pains, persistent *Lajin* helps a meditator sit cross-legged more easily.

There is still no telling exactly how many diseases can be improved by practicing *Lajin* in Reclining Posture.

2: SQUATTING POSTURE

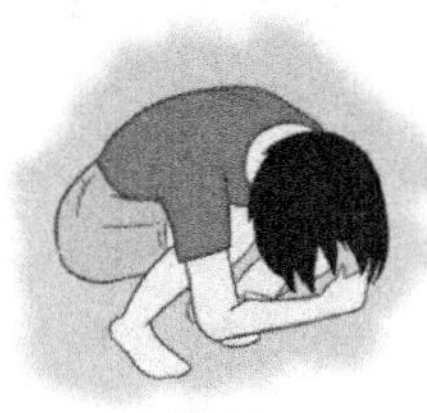
蹲式拉筋

This is the oldest natural stretching exercise. It is also called "baby hugging"—similar to the posture of a baby in its mother's womb.

It clears multiple meridians along the legs and feet, including the Liver, Spleen, Kidney, Stomach, Gall Bladder, and Urinary Bladder Meridians. It's a great stretch for:

- Heels
- Ankles
- Calves
- Knees
- Buttocks
- Waistlines

The bent knees, hips, and waist are a good massage for the internal organs as well.

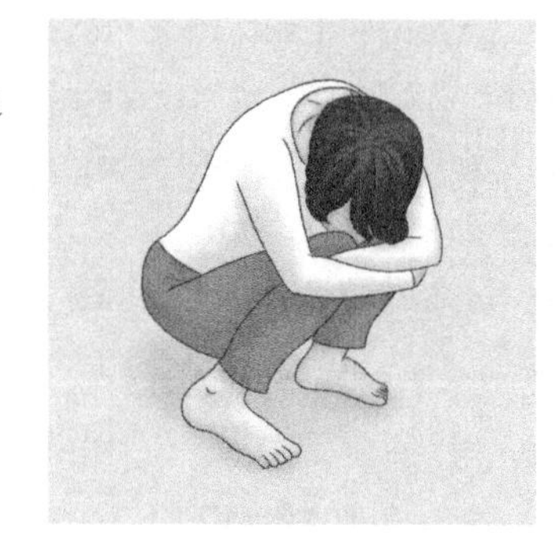

Simply squat down on the ground for five to forty minutes.

Beginners may find it easier to squat with their feet spread apart. The level of difficulty increases when your feet are closer together. For best effects, try to squat as low as possible, put your feet together, lower your head, and hold your arms around your knees.

It is more difficult to squat with bare feet, but the effect is better. Chinese people used to do many things squatting down: they ate, chatted, and even held meetings in this posture, as can be spotted in many old movies.

Yet, influenced by waves of modernization, even squat toilets were replaced by seated ones. Passing stool in a squat is natural—it clears meridian blockages and massages the intestines and internal organs, contributing to a better bowel movement. The seated toilet may look graceful and comfortable, but it deprives us of natural massage and stretching. No wonder more and more people now have lower back and leg pain and find it difficult to squat down.

Benefits of Squatting Posture

Squatting Posture is a carpet-bombing exercise. Tendons that aren't fully stretched during Reclining Posture are targeted when squatting. It helps your:

- Heels
- Ankles
- Calves
- Knees
- Hips
- Hip joints
- Tail bone
- Waist
- Back
- Chest
- Shoulders
- Neck

It also stimulates bowel movements, enhances *qi* and blood circulation, and clears all major meridians. Squatting Position also improves:

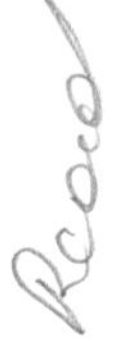

- Hemorrhoids
- Arthritis
- Diabetes
- Hypertension
- Constipation
- Gastroenteritis
- Heart disease
- Prostate disorders
- Gynecological disorders
- Lower back and leg pain

3: STANDING ON A BOARD POSTURE

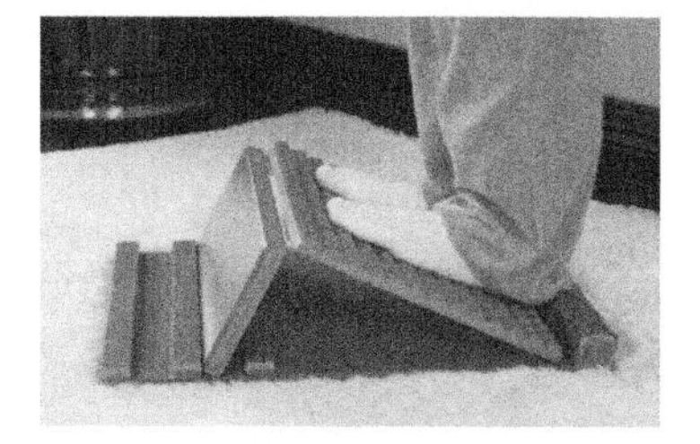

1) Stand on a sloping, standing board with graded levels of difficulty.
2) Raise your toes, try to stand up straight, and keep your balance.
3) Hold your hands high above your head if possible. If necessary, you can also place them behind your back or let them hang down naturally
4) Stand in this posture for ten to sixty minutes.

In the beginning, you may feel pain and soreness. You might experience swelling.

If so, you can ease into the practice by tilting your hips back for balance. With practice, your hips will return to their natural position, and you will be able to stretch longer. Then you can increase the level of difficulty. This *Lajin* posture stretches almost all your major tendons and meridians: including your calves, buttocks, waist, and kidneys—but especially along the soles, heels, ankles, and backs of your feet.

Benefits of Standing on a Board Posture

As you age, your legs will show signs of aging first.

Three *yin* and three *yang* meridians run along the feet and legs. These meridians are the most susceptible to cold and are blocked the earliest, and many toxins are deposited in the feet due to gravity.

Stretching on a *Lajin* stand board thoroughly cleans many acupoints on the feet and the calves, which can't be stretched well in other *Lajin* postures. It can help relieve:

- Foot pain
- Leg pain
- Waist pain
- Diabetes
- Hypertension
- Heart disease
- Prostate disorders
- Liver and kidney problems
- Strokes
- Cancer

The *Lajin* board is very small, and it takes very little space. It is a very convenient tool for health preservation, both at home and in the office. Some people stand on the board chatting, reading, watching TV, or even working on a computer.

4: STANDING POSTURE

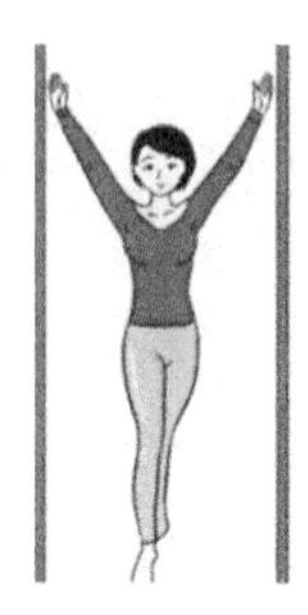 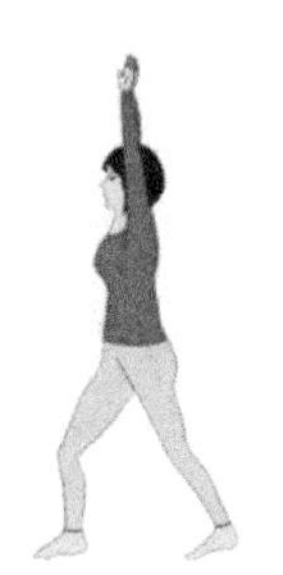 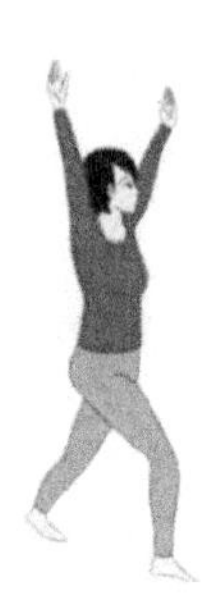

1) Stand in a doorframe, hold the sides of it with your hands, and stretch your arms as much as possible.
2) Place one foot forward to do a bow step.
3) Straighten the other foot as much as possible.
4) Keep your heels on the ground.
5) Keep your upper body parallel to the doorframe, with your head upright. Your eyes should look straight ahead.
6) Do this for five to eight minutes. Then switch legs.

Benefits of Standing Posture

Lajin in Standing Posture acts on the meridians around: the shoulders, back, and legs. It helps with:

- Neck pain
- Frozen shoulders
- Back pain
- Mammary gland diseases
- Hyperthyroidism
- Lung diseases

The Urinary Bladder Meridian at the back of the calves is also stretched.

5: Y-SHAPED POSTURE

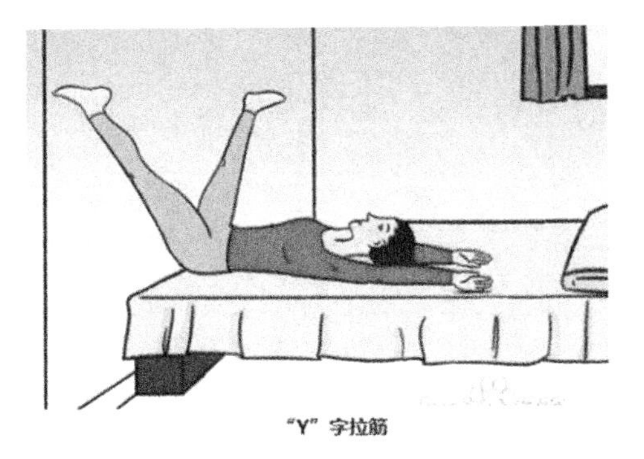

"Y" 字拉筋

1) Lie on the ground or on a bed.
2) One leg should be held down by another person.
3) Spread your other leg horizontally as much as you can.
4) Stay in this posture for three to thirty minutes, then switch legs.

Alternately:

1) Lie on a bed or a mat with your buttocks pressed against the wall.
2) Raise your legs and spread them as far apart as possible, in a capital-letter Y shape.
3) Stay in this posture for three to thirty minutes.

Benefits of Y-Shaped Posture:

- Y-Shaped Posture helps with lower back and sacrum pain.
- It powerfully dredges the Liver, Spleen, and Kidney Meridians along the inner side of each leg, which enhances the functions of the three corresponding organs.
- It can make your legs slimmer as well.

6: NECK *LAJIN*

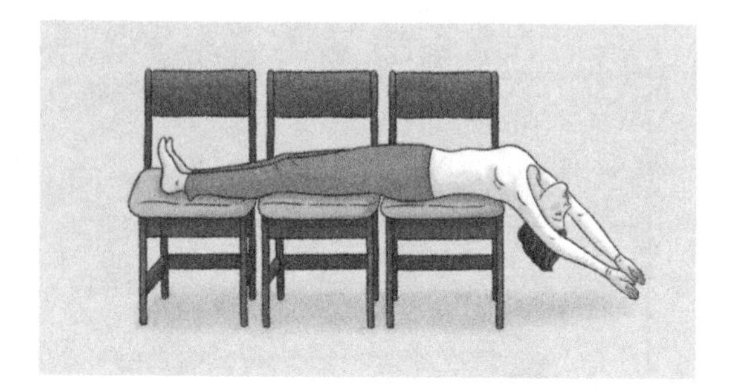

1) Lie flat on a bed, chairs, or a *Lajin* bench.
2) Move your head, neck, and upper shoulders off the edge.
3) Let them hang down naturally.
4) Stretch your arms as far backward as possible.
5) Stay in this posture for five to eight minutes.

Benefits of Neck *Lajin*

Neck *Lajin* relieves diseases related to your neck and chest vertebrae, shoulders, and upper back. It's useful for treating:

- Headaches
- Dizziness
- Asthma
- Rhinitis
- Cataracts
- Glaucoma
- Blindness
- Scoliosis
- Neck stiffness
- Chest tightness
- Frozen shoulders
- Thyroid disease
- Cardiovascular and cerebrovascular disease
- Hyperplasia of mammary glands

When you hang your head in an inverted position, more *qi* and blood flow to your brain, eyes, nose, and ears, healing your head and face. By hanging down some of your chest vertebras, you relieve diseases related to your heart and lungs.

Reminder: If you experience dizziness or suffer from hypertension, cardiovascular problems, or cerebrovascular disease, it is advisable to do this exercise gradually.

7: *LAJIN* WHILE SLEEPING

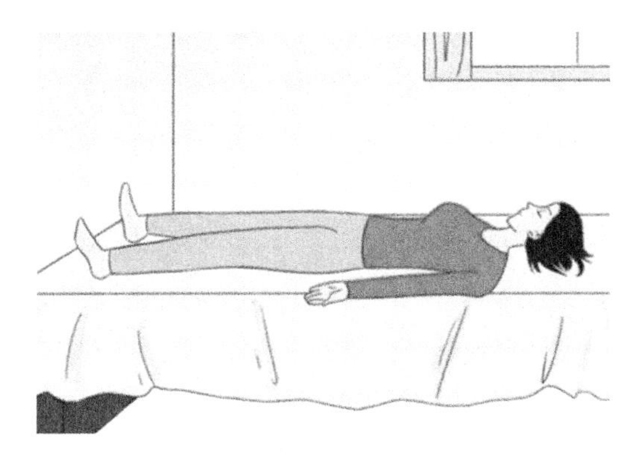

It is also known as "bone setting during sleep".

Sleep on a hard bed or a hard mattress, preferably without a pillow.

This will stretch your neck and your entire spine, realigning your bones. It can be practiced in any sleeping pose.

Because people's heads tend to lean forward for a long time when working, neck problems are common. *Lajin* during sleep reverses the direction of gravity. It is gentle, yet effective. If you always use a pillow, you may need a few nights to get used to it.

Many people who gain instant relief from *Lajin* or bone setting find their challenges reoccur later on. They haven't changed their habits—they still sit on soft couches and sleep on soft mattresses. Sitting and sleeping on mats or wooden beds are traditional practices that are unfortunately no longer popular in China. However, these traditions are still very much alive and well in Korean and Japanese cultures.

People think hard beds cause them pain, but the firm nature actually acts against the body's weight—in a natural manner—to realign the bones. If a hard bed isn't available, simply sleep on the ground, as long as it isn't cold or damp. We absorb energy from the Earth when we sleep. Sleeping on the ground, especially on the ground floor, is much healthier.

In short, sitting and sleeping on hard surfaces is natural stretching and bone setting.

Benefits of *Lajin* During Sleep

It is safe and natural. Stretching happens naturally during sleep, and the force comes from the body's own weight. Make it a habit. Minor vertebrae dislocations can be naturally realigned.

It is a simple diagnostic method to locate health problems: where there is pain, there is a problem.

Antique Chinese furniture was square-shaped because it enabled a person to keep their body straight—and naturally stretch. People who watch TV or chat while curling in comfortable couches or soft beds for long periods of time are more likely to have scoliosis, waist pain, knee pain, dislocations of bones, stiff tendons, and blocked meridians. In meditation, one of the requirements is to sit straight. It helps to keep the bones aligned and tendons supple. This will eventually help to clear meridians.

Duration and Intensity

It isn't possible to set absolute standards for *Lajin*. Each person differs in age, physique, and health condition. Patients and the elderly can't be expected to stretch properly the first time. What is important is to stretch until you feel soreness, numbness, pain, and swelling.

Countless clinical studies show *Lajin* is more effective when practiced for up to twenty minutes. It's much better than two ten-minute sessions. Adding seven to twenty-two-pound sandbags to each leg makes it even more effective.

Some people feel excruciating pain right away, revealing severe health problems. These people need to persist with *Lajin*, and gradually stretch longer and add weights. For those who practice yoga or dance regularly, ten minutes of *Lajin* isn't a big deal. Once you extend it to thirty to forty minutes per leg, they will begin to feel unpleasant things. They sweat, fart, belch, and feel a need to void their bowels. This is a good sign.

The record time of *Lajin* in Reclining Posture is two hours a day—stretching each leg for one hour, with twenty-two-pound sandbags on each leg. The result: a man's gout, hypertension, and heart disease were healed. He stopped taking all of his medications.

It should be noted: *Lajin*'s duration is only counted after pain, swelling, soreness, numbness, and tightness are felt. This is when the self-healing mechanism begins its work. It is no use stretching for a long time if you feel none of those sensations. If you stop stretching after feeling a little pain or numbness, or just lie down comfortably, how could it possibly work? We strongly advise using the *Lajin* bench to speed up the effects, while remaining safe.

IMPORTANT NOTES:

1. When practicing *Lajin* outside, avoid wind and chills.
2. When practicing inside, avoid electric fans or air conditioners. Sweating during *Lajin* is beneficial, so don't cool down deliberately.
3. Your waist and knees should never be exposed because your pores open up during *Lajin*.
4. Wear long-sleeved shirts and pants to stay warm.

5. For better and faster effects, stretch with more weights for a longer time. If you dance, practice yoga, or have a very flexible body, you can stretch each leg over the above recommended times.
6. If the sole of your foot can't touch the ground during Reclining Posture, you can slightly move your lowered leg outward to ease the pain. Once your stretching improves, move both of your legs close together to avoid splayed feet.
7. Women can practice *Lajin* at any point in their cycle. *Lajin* practice during your period helps with menstrual pain.
8. Stay attentive when doing *Lajin*. When you feel pain, add in some *Paida*. If *Lajin* is difficult, slap your joints, hands, and feet.

CAUTION:

People with hypertension, heart disease, and critical illnesses, and people who are elderly or weak, should take it slowly. Pain increases your pulse rate and blood pressure. These are ultimately good reactions, but you need to pace yourself. You can prop your head up with a small pillow to avoid blood rushing to your brain.

If you have extreme reactions, stop for a while and slap heavily on your inner elbows and your Neiguan Acupoints near your wrists.

12

REASONS TO ATTEND *PAIDALAJIN* WORKSHOPS

Since *PaidaLajin* is so simple and effective, I initially assumed everyone would be able to practice using my books, videos, and websites.

However, few people are disciplined enough to persist in intensive and persistent practice. Therefore, we resorted to organizing *PaidaLajin* self-healing workshops. We have been receiving enthusiastic responses from all over the world. We held the first workshop in Beijing on November 6, 2010. Since then, we have organized several hundred workshops in Beijing, Shanghai, Shenzhen, and other cities in the Chinese mainland, as well as in Hong Kong, Macau, Taiwan, India, Indonesia, Singapore, Malaysia, Germany, Switzerland, Bulgaria, Holland, Australia, Canada, the US, South Africa, and many other countries and territories. Thousands of people have attended and greatly benefited from the workshops. It is expected such workshops will be conducted at many other places in the future.

Prior to the workshops, despite studies, many people questioned its effectiveness. Because self-healing testimonials came from all corners of the world, we were accused of announcing only the successful ones. Voices of doubt persisted after we published the effective improvement rates of various diseases through *PaidaLajin* at the workshops.

We welcome experts and medical institutions to come to our workshops to perform tests, take measurements, and record observations using general acknowledged indicators, methods, and devices of their preference.

Even using the most conservative statistics, the effective rates of *PaidaLajin* in resolving various health problems during workshops exceed 80%.

The most prominent effects from the workshops:

- Insomnia
- Diabetes
- Hypertension
- Heart Disease
- Knee Pain
- Frozen Shoulders
- Neck Stiffness and Pain
- Lower Back and Leg Pain
- Prostate Disorders
- Gynecological Disorders

Almost all workshop participants have complex diseases. Almost everyone experiences improvement.

Some people practice for half a year, along with other treatments such as medication, surgery, massage, acupressure, acupuncture, bone setting, or skin-scraping before attending a workshop. However, they make far greater improvements at the workshop.

1. *PaidaLajin* may appear simple, but changing the Heart is difficult.

Confidence, determination, perseverance, patience, repentance, and gratitude come from the Heart. The power of the Heart is a decisive factor in self-healing. After it's tapped into, two simple exercises reap both physical and psychological benefits. Workshop participants are taught the principles of nursing the Heart by coaches, who assist and guide them whenever problems arise.

The art of healing the Heart has always been passed down from master to disciple on a one-to-one basis. This is the true significance of the workshop.

2. ***PaidaLajin* at home isn't as intense as it is during the workshop.**

Workshop activities are conducted in an environment isolated from the outside world, thus enabling participants to fully concentrate. *PaidaLajin* is practiced at least four to five hours a day using the carpet-bombing strategy. No body part is spared. This is difficult to achieve in the home environment. The disparity in intensity is even greater. Some participants find that ten minutes of *Paida* in the workshop is better than a one hour at home. The same goes for *Lajin*. This is especially true for men, who are usually more afraid of pain and normally do not use heavy *Paida* on themselves.

3. **The workshop provides a vegetarian diet and other benefits.**

Eating less than usual is encouraged by the coaches. The program also includes fasting, meditation, meditative jogging, emotional sharing, and more. Each of these activities produces unique benefits in nursing the Heart. When combined with *PaidaLajin*, the healing effect is even better. Such resources and this atmosphere can rarely be found in the home environment.

4. **The proper use of *Lajin* benches greatly enhances healing.**

Lajin is practiced several times a day during the workshop, and it is taught and moderated by the coaches. It may be hard to convince yourself to practice long enough on your own.

Doing *Lajin* with chairs and a doorframe is only a temporary substitute. In order to gain better healing effects, it is a must to do *Lajin* on a proper *Lajin* bench. This is especially true for those with chronic or critical illnesses. And for anyone using a *Lajin* bench, if the raised leg is not strapped tightly against the pole or the lowered leg is not weighed down with sandbags, the healing effect is discounted.

5. **The positive atmosphere (the *Qi* field.)**

The feelings created during the workshop are unimaginable to those practicing *PaidaLajin* at home. Practicing *PaidaLajin* in a large group creates a very encouraging resonance effect. Laypersons, experienced doctors, and health specialists are treated equally at the workshop. Peer pressure and mutual motivation drive participants to put in maximum efforts. By witnessing improvements in fellow participants, you are inspired to persevere more intensely for longer periods of time.

When many people practicing intensive *PaidaLajin* together, a person can experience and witness inspiring self-healing miracles every day.

- A patient with leg pain might walk without crutches and even run.
- Someone who has been deaf for decades might hear sound again.
- Diabetic or hypertensive patient's blood glucose or blood pressure levels become normal over time—without medication or insulin.

If you're in doubt, it might change your mind.

6. **Healing reactions are better dealt with at a workshop.**

At home, people might not know how to deal with pain, numbness, soreness, swelling, rashes, insomnia, itchiness, nausea, vomiting, coughing, dizziness, irregular heartbeats, chest tightness, crying, and old injuries and illnesses resurfacing.

Participants are also taught how to lessen the side effects by slapping their inner elbows and *Neiguan* Acupoints instead of going to the emergency room.

7. **The toxic side effects of drugs are reduced during the workshop.**

Doctors of Chinese and Western Medicine know medication has toxic side effects. There are even specific terms in the West:

drug-induced and iatrogenic diseases. Surgery, chemotherapy, and other treatments can lead to new diseases. At our self-healing workshops, many participants voluntarily reduce or stop their medication. This reduces the risks of drug-induced diseases.

Note: *PaidaLajin* is not a medical therapy. Participants should talk to their doctors before reducing or stopping medications.

8. There are mutual *Paida* sessions.

People who have difficulty with *Paida* receive a lot of assistance at the workshops. Also, many body parts are hard for anyone to reach.

The people at the workshops are caring and positive, enabling better physical and spiritual interactions. These external measures help to heal the Heart.

9. It's easier to learn.

The coaches and the other participants will help you learn the practice more quickly and easily.

Post-Workshop Reports

The workshops are a good starting place, but *PaidaLajin* doesn't end when you go home. The goal isn't temporary healing or fixing conditions you have at the time. It's a life-long effort to change your habits and mindset.

Fortunately, most people make genuine lifestyle changes after they complete their workshop.

13

IMPORTANT ACUPOINTS

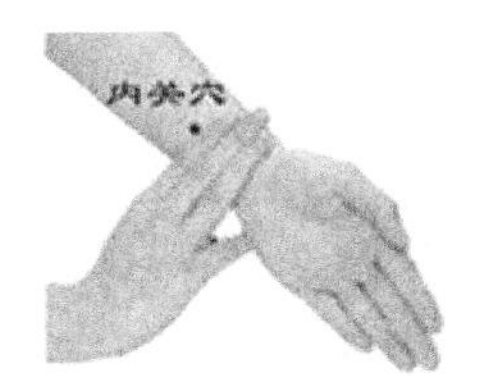

Neiguan Acupoints

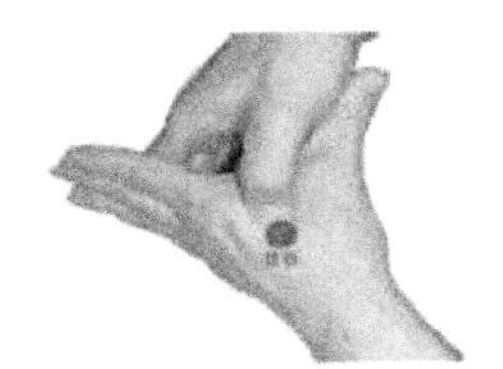

Hegu Acupoints

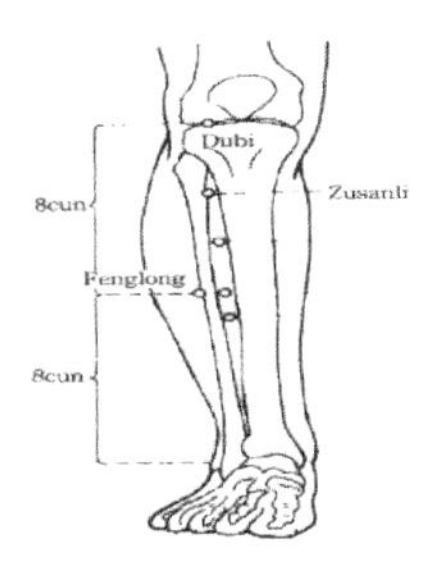

Zusanli Acupoints

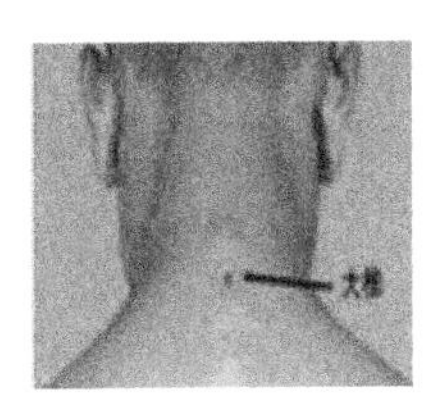

Dazhui Acupoints

14

THE GENERAL *PAIDA* SEQUENCE

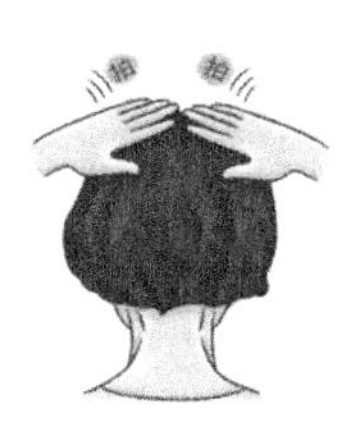
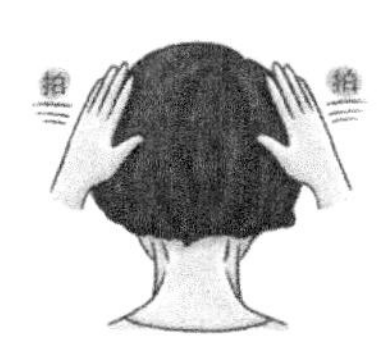
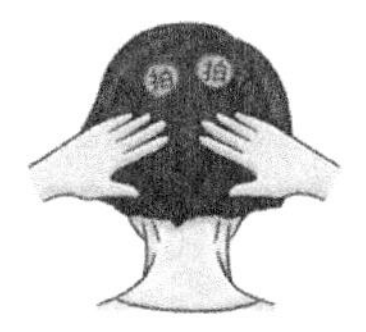
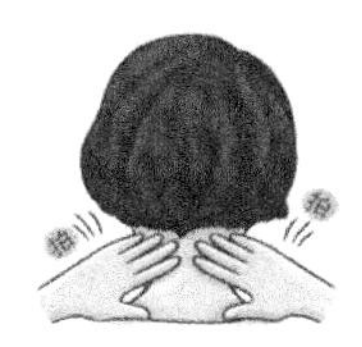

Universal Regions and the Head

Theoretically, all body parts can be slapped. Normally, *Paida* follows a top-down sequence. When sick, a person will want to identify blocked meridians.

There are fourteen meridians in the body—twelve standard meridians, and the Ren and Du meridians along the median part of the torso. All illness originates from blockages of these fourteen meridians, whether they be mosquito bites, tumors, insomnia, or constipation. Normally, multiple meridians are blocked in a sick person. Unblocking the fourteen meridians will cure everything.

However, many people do not have enough time to slap their entire body. They tend to look for key areas related to their specific symptoms. We recommend slapping the head and four universal regions, which basically covers all fourteen meridians.

The four universal regions:

- Elbows (front and back)
- Knees (front, back, left, and right sides)
- Hands (front and back sides)
- Feet (top, bottom, left, and right sides)

When slapping elbows or knees, thoroughly slap all four sides.

1. Place one of your hands on a knee. *Paida* the back of that hand and your fingers with the palm of the other hand.
2. When you *Paida* the feet, thoroughly slap the inner and outer sides of the ankles. Then move to the tops and soles of the feet.
3. Slap each area for fifteen minutes or more. Make it a habit to slap at least one universal region each day.

The Head

After completing the universal regions, *Paida* the entire head, including:

- The top, left, right, front, and back sides
- Neck
- Closed eyes
- Cheeks
- Nose
- Mouth
- Ears

Slapping the head helps to relieve all chronic diseases. It's particularly effective for healing:

- Headaches
- Insomnia
- Diseases of the five-sensory organs
- Cardiovascular disease
- Alzheimer's disease

This is because every *yang* meridian goes up to the head. For instance, Liver opens into the eyes; Kidney opens into the ears; Lung opens into the nose; Spleen opens into the mouth; and Heart opens into the tongue. Thus, slapping the entire head also heals internal organ disorders.

The Eight Weak Corners

The *Huang Di Nei Jing* dubbed the following the Eight Weak Corners:

- Armpits
- Groin
- Inner elbows
- The popliteal fossa (back of the knees)

They are mostly likely to accumulate cold-dampness, toxins, and wastes. Clearing these areas is a shortcut to healing. But the armpits and the groin aren't included in the universal regions for *Paida*, because they are less convenient to slap and the pain is greater. You may reject *Paida* altogether if you feel too much pain during your initial experience. However, at our workshops, these are key targets.

After finishing the head and universal regions, slap the armpits and groin. Then slap:

- Your entire four limbs
- Chest
- Back
- Abdomen
- Buttocks

In other words, carpet bomb your entire body.

15

MAINTENANCE AFTER YOU'RE HEALTHY

Paida is practiced in a top-down order for maintenance purposes:

1. Head

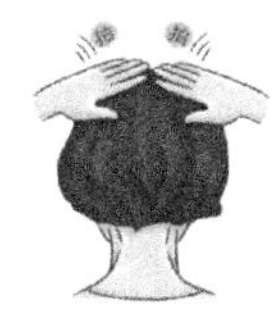
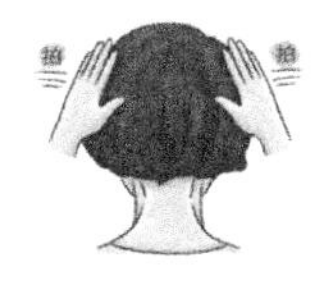
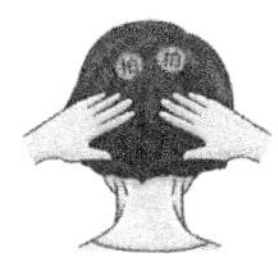
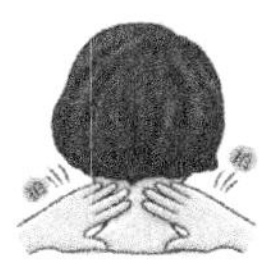

Slap the top, left, and right side of the head. Then move to the front and back sides. You may use one hand or both. Slapping the back of the head with one hand is more convenient. Then move on to slap the back of your neck, closed eyes, cheeks, mouth, and ears. You may feel warmth or numbness at the perineum, which is between your legs, or on the soles of your feet during this time.

2. Shoulders

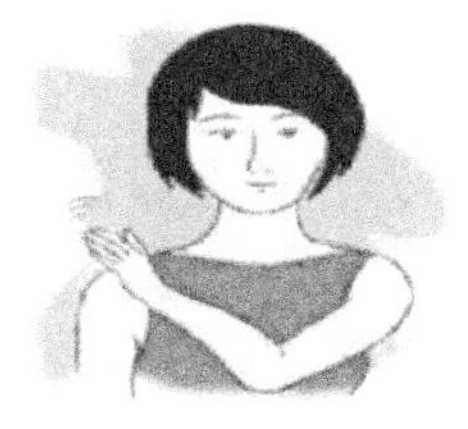

Use the left hand to slap the right shoulder and vice versa. Slap the front, back, top, and outer sides of both shoulders.

3. Arms, Armpits, and Inner Ribs

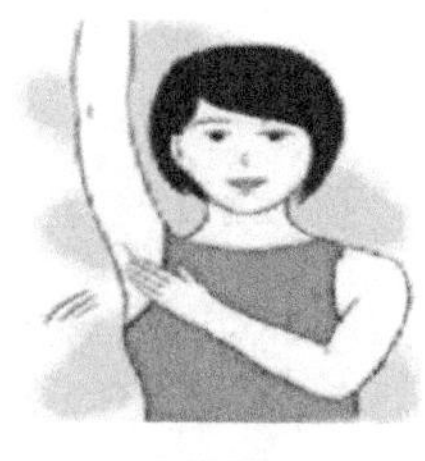

4. Elbows

Slap on the inner side of each elbow, which covers the Heart, Pericardium, and Lung Meridians. Then slap on the outer side, which includes the Large Intestine, San Jiao (Triple Warmer), and Small Intestine Meridians.

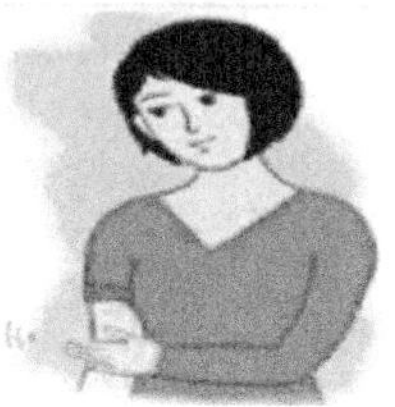

5. Back of Hands

Put one hand on your knee with the back of the hand facing up, then slap hard with the other hand. Switch hands afterward.

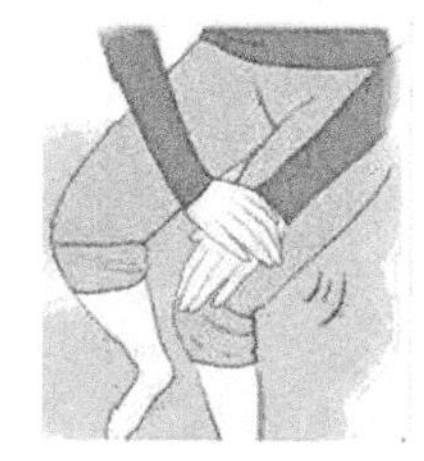

6. Buttocks

Include hip joints and surrounding areas.

7. Thighs

Slap the inner and outer sides of one thigh with both hands, and then move on to slap the other thigh.

8. Abdomen and Groin

Slap with palms, chop with the sides of hands, or beat with fists.

9. Knees

Slap the front of your knees with both hands, covering an entire kneecap with your palm. Next, slap the inner and outer sides of a knee with both hands. Then move on to slap the other knee. Lastly, *Paida* the back of the knees, which may be done by opening the legs while being seated, or you can put one foot on top of a chair while standing.

People can also *Paida* each other in a group if this proves difficult.

10. Feet

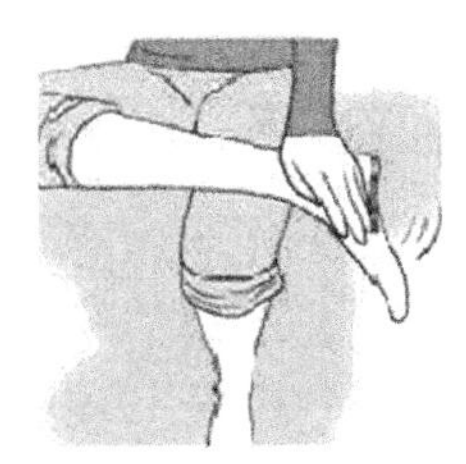

This includes the tops and soles of the feet, the inner and outer sides of the ankles, and the surrounding areas.

CAUTION: Those about to undergo surgery may recover through *Paida* instead, sparing them an invasive procedure. For better healing, combine *Paida* with *Lajin*.

SELF-HELP *PAIDA* AND MUTUAL *PAIDA*

It is better to slap both yourself and others.

Self-help *Paida* is effective, because the power of the Heart—your greatest power—is mobilized. Mutual *Paida* is a good if you struggle with implementation, especially due to illness. Mutual *Paida* creates a more positive atmosphere and a stronger energy field, and some people do need help from others. Even when we primarily do it on our own, it's easier if others help us with:

- Our back
- Armpits
- Shoulders
- Backs of the knees
- Hind side of the legs
- Other inconvenient locations

Many people are overly protective of themselves—they *Paida* too gently for *sha* to appear, which leads them to assume they're in good health. This can mask grave illnesses. For some people, it reveals weak heart and kidney functions, a lack of strength, and weak willpower, which tends to be more common in men. More often than not, when others slap them a bit harder, *sha* comes out.

People who play year-round sports or practice *qi* gong assume they are quite healthy. *Sha* does not appear easily on them during regular *Paida*. However, when they slap each other, each and every one of them are covered with *sha*. Despite how horrendous it looks, many old injuries and past diseases are revealed and uprooted once and for all. This can even untie "knots" deep in our hearts that have tortured us for decades.

Duration and Intensity

Generally speaking, there needs to be moderate pain with *Paida* or it won't work. You will slap each body region for five to sixty minutes each time. Severe symptoms will require more strength and time. Five minutes is considered effective. The self-healing mechanism will not be fully activated without some pain.

During our seven-day *PaidaLajin* self-healing workshops, participants:

- Slap for six hours
- Stretch for an hour
- *Paida* all major body parts

It takes up to fifteen days to complete a thorough, all-body *Paida*. Back home, it is difficult to slap and stretch so hard and for so long. You can adjust according to your health and other factors. Extend the time when it's possible. For maintenance, after you're healthy:

1. *Paida* the entire head and the universal regions for half to a full hour each day.
2. During normal illness, *Paida* the universal regions and illness-related areas for one to three hours.
3. If you are seriously ill, *Paida* your entire body multiple times.

PaidaLajin is simple, but to grasp the essence of it, it's best to attend a workshop to most effectively learn the techniques, duration, intensity, and power of the Heart. Up to now, we have not found a better way for people to learn and benefit from *PaidaLajin* than attending a workshop.

If you can attach the same importance to your health as you do to games, sports, and dining, you will find you have time for *PaidaLajin*.

Paida a body region thoroughly before moving on to the next region. For example, pick an inner elbow, the top of your head, or the front side of your knee. Practice *Paida* there for five to sixty minutes.

Thorough *Paida*

Paida until *sha* comes out of the slapped area.

Continue until:

- The *sha* disappears
- The pain is reduced
- The skin is broken and blood or bodily fluid seeps out

When covering a large region, focus on an area the size of your palm. Slap for five to sixty minutes. Then move to the next area.

1. It's best to *Paida* yourself on easy-to-reach body parts. Help others with regions that are harder to access.
2. Take turns between using your hands and *Paida* sticks. Use a stick when you feel tired or when *sha* doesn't easily appear. In cold weather, use a *Paida* stick over clothing.
3. Do not stop halfway during *Paida*. It's best to slap a body part thoroughly. When the *sha* disappears, start a second round.
4. Some people self-heal after a round of thorough *Paida* all over their body. However, many patients need multiple rounds of carpet-bombing *Paida* for a full recovery. Adjust the areas and frequency to suit your needs.
5. Focus on universal or other specific regions.

6. It is more effective to do *Paida* and one to three *Lajin* sessions per day.
7. You can do *Lajin* without the standard *Lajin* bench or sandbags, and put down your raised leg when it feels sore, numb, painful, or if there's swelling. It's more efficient and effective on the special bench, using ten to forty-four-pound sandbags. Continue to stretch after feeling unpleasant sensations.
8. Gentle *Paida* requires at least moderate pain. However, it will take longer. You may have to slap one region for thirty minutes to two hours.

Helping Others

Some patients are unable to do *PaidaLajin* on their own. Family members, relatives, and friends can help them.

1. Slap the inner elbows and the backs of their hands.
2. Move to their knees and feet.
3. Continue to their head, belly, and entire four limbs.
4. Slap each region for five to sixty minutes.
5. To relieve more severe symptoms, *Paida* longer and for additional rounds.
6. Slap all over the body during several sessions.

Bed-Ridden Patients

1. Help them lift up one leg to stretch, since they can't use a *Lajin* bench.
2. The stretching is effective as long as the patient feels soreness, numbness, pain, or swelling.

3. The duration of stretching varies with each individual's physique and health condition.
4. You can start with several seconds.
5. Gradually it can be extended to several minutes or longer.
6. When healing reactions occur, shorten the time and reduce the intensity of *PaidaLajin*.
7. Have them rest and drink ginger and jujube tea.

16

STEPS FOR SPECIFIC DISORDERS, DISEASES, AND CONDITIONS

Remember, to truly gain and retain health, you must consistently *Paida* your entire body. However, you can place more focus on acute problems. This alphabetical list gives you more details.

ACUTE LIVER PAIN AND GALL BLADDER PAIN

Slap along the Gall Bladder Meridian on the outer side of each leg, inner elbows, and the *Neiguan* Acupoints.

ABDOMINAL PAIN

1. Slap the *Zusanli* Acupoints, *Neiguan* Acupoints, and the abdomen.
2. Do *Lajin* in Squatting Posture.
3. Stretch on a *Lajin* bench.

ADDICTION (SEE CRITICAL DISEASES)

AIDS (SEE CRITICAL DISEASES)

ALZHEIMER'S DISEASE

Alzheimer's symptoms appear in almost all elderly people, although it sometimes other forms of dementia.

Normally, dementia patients suffer from many other chronic diseases, including:

- Organ Malfunction
- Brain Syndromes
- Issues with Limbs
- Disorders of the Five Sensory Organs
- Deficient Memory
- Speech Impairment
- Mobility issues

Some elderly people have received gentle *Paida* in a nursing home in San Francisco. They have shown improvements in:

- Memory
- Speech
- Hearing
- Appetite
- Mobility
- Elimination

1. *Paida* the universal regions (elbows, knees, hands, and feet), particularly their inner elbows and the back of their hands.
2. In the beginning, just slap on the top, left, right, front, and back sides of their head and neck.
3. After the patient adjusts to *Paida*, slap their eyes, ears, cheeks, and mouth as well.
4. Try to engage and guide dementia patients into group slapping and stretching games.
5. DO NOT forcefully straighten the legs of patients with very stiff muscles.
6. Begin raising and stretching the legs alternately while the patient lies flat in bed. It is working as long as the patient feels pain.

So no need of special bench. Bed or chair will do

7. Gradually extend the time and lift the legs higher. And then move on to use the *Lajin* bench.
8. Slap each region for five to sixty minutes each time.
9. To relieve more severe symptoms, *Paida* longer and for additional rounds.

Elderly patients with normal mobility and cognition can practice self-healing.

ANKYLOSING SPONDYLITIS (SEE CRITICAL DISEASES)

Stretch more and slap along the entire spine. Practice the wall-hitting exercise to stimulate the back and spine.

AUTISM

Autism usually starts very young.

1. Encourage autistic children to play the *Paida* Game.
2. They can do regular wall hitting, tie qiang gong, and waist swirling exercises in a group.
3. Gradually go from gentle to heavier *Paida*.
4. Pat the universal regions (elbows, knees, hands, and feet.)
5. Focus on patting the four limbs, head, hands, and feet for five to sixty minutes each.
6. To relieve more severe symptoms, *Paida* longer and for additional rounds.
7. Do not panic when you see *sha*, lumps, and swelling.
8. Provide ginger and jujube tea daily.
9. Do daily warm-water footbaths in 104° F water (40° C).
10. Stretch one to three times a day.

11. Gradually extend the time to over thirty minutes per leg each time.

Paida on a child appears cruel, and some people can't make themselves do it. However, when you pat a kid with loving care, in spite of *sha*, pain, crying, and swelling, it is beneficial to the child. It is true love.

BREAST CANCER AND MAMMARY GLAND HYPERPLASIA

Globally, doctors prescribe annual breast screenings for women. Many women with diseases of the breast also suffer from varying degrees of depression, which is a form of Heart disease. In short, emotional problems are at the root of breast diseases. They are caused by blockages in the Heart and Pericardium Meridians.

Even for a woman diagnosed with breast cancer or mammary gland hyperplasia, the disease names are still misleading. Cancer and hyperplasia are the "fruits" of problems within the patient's internal organs, especially the heart.

1. Slap the universal regions (knees, hands, and feet.)
2. Slap all around the breasts, particularly the outer sides adjacent to the armpits, and the entire armpits.
3. Move on to slap the chest and back.
4. Continue until *sha*, lumps, swelling, and pain disappear. The process can be quite painful.
5. Slap the head, groin, four limbs, abdomen, and buttocks.
6. Carpet bomb the entire body.
7. Stretch one to three times a day, and gradually extend the time up to thirty minutes per leg each time.
8. Add sandbags weighing 6.5–33 pounds on each leg.

9. Drink ginger and jujube tea.
10. Do daily warm-water footbaths in 104° F water (40° C).
11. It's best to attend a *PaidaLajin* workshop.
12. Try meditative jogging, waist swirling, wall hitting, and *tie qiang gong* (see video tutorials on the English website.)
13. Slap each region for five to sixty minutes each time.
14. To relieve more severe symptoms, *Paida* longer and for additional rounds.

Slapping the breasts is an ideal way to screen and prevent breast cancer.

BURNS AND SPRAINS

1. Slap around the burn or sprain, and then move to the injured area.
2. Slap the painful area and the matching spot on the other side of the body.

   For example, if your big toe on your left foot is injured, also slap the thumb of your right hand. Your left elbow matches with your right knee, and your left shoulder matches the right side of your groin.

CAUTION: DO NOT slap on body parts with open wounds or fractured bones.

CANCER (SEE CHRONIC DISEASES)

CHILDREN (SEE PEDIATRIC DISORDERS)

CHRONIC DISEASES

All chronic diseases are complex diseases. That is to say, a chronic disease is an aggregated manifestation of several or dozens of underlying health problems. These include:

- Cancer
- Diabetes
- Hypertension
- Heart disease
- Endocrine disorders
- Neurological disorders
- Problems with the liver, spleen, stomach, kidneys, large, and small intestines

The disease names vary, but they are basically labels for particular symptoms. As long as new indicators are detected with medical instruments, more and more new disease names will be created.

Treating Chronic Diseases

Since they are complex diseases, all internal organs are compromised, and all fourteen major meridians are suffering from blockages, to varying degrees.

1. Stretch on a *Lajin* bench.
2. Slap the universal regions (elbows, knees, hands, and feet.)
3. Follow with the entire head, all four limbs, and all joints and regions of the body.
4. Include the chest, back, belly, groin, armpits, and buttocks.
5. During the process of *PaidaLajin* for chronic diseases, it is best to fast for three to four days.
6. People with weak *qi* and insufficient blood supply can also try fasting.

7. Drink some ginger and jujube tea to replenish *qi* and blood flow.

CHRONIC FATIGUE SYNDROME

- Headaches
- Insomnia
- Irritation
- Mood swings
- Unexplained fatigue
- Low energy
- Waist pain
- Soreness
- Stiffness
- Fear of Extreme Temperatures

1. Do *Lajin* in Reclining Posture twice a day. Stretch each leg for ten to fifty minutes each time and add twenty-two to forty-pound sandbags to each leg.
2. *Paida* the universal regions (elbows, knees, hands, and feet.)
3. Slap the head, inner elbows, *Neiguan* Acupoints, and the top and sides of your head.
4. Slap along all four limbs.
5. Do meditation, wall hitting, waist swirling, *tie qiang gong*, and breathing exercises.
6. Zen jog for thirty to sixty minutes each morning.
7. Do meditative standing for ten to sixty minutes each morning when the sun is rising.
8. Massage your waist regularly. Press your hands on your waist and rub down to the lower end of your spine. Repeat 100–200 times each morning and evening.

9. You can also gently pat your waist.
10. Do daily warm-water footbaths in 104° F water (40° C). Stop when your back starts to sweat. Add your hands and forearms to the water when possible.
11. Massage your feet during and after the footbath, or *Paida* the feet afterwards.
12. Receive acupressure, acupuncture, chiropractic, or other holistic treatments. There may be dislocated joints along your spine.
13. Avoid overeating. Eat until your stomach is 50–70% full. You can also fast for three to seven days each month.
14. Don't eat a lot of meat. It takes too much energy to digest. Add more grains into your diet.
15. Go to sleep before midnight. The best time to go to sleep is between 9:00–11:00 p.m. Early to bed and early to rise. It's good to take a short nap around noon.
16. Do not drink too much alcohol. Drink moderately. Too much drinking is harmful to the liver, spleen, and kidneys.
17. Quit smoking. Smoking is bad for your lungs, and nicotine slows down your blood flow. It contributes to high blood lipids, blood glucose, and blood pressure. It can also lead to poor erectile function.
18. Avoid having too much sex. Similar to tasty food, having too much is counterproductive.

COMMON COLDS: FEVERS, FATIGUE, HEADACHES, AND COUGHING

1. Slap the inner elbows and *Dazhui* Acupoints (at the protruding juncture of the neck and shoulders.)

2. Slap each for thirty minutes.
3. Go gradually from soft to heavy *Paida*.
4. Use soft, caring, and attentive patting on a child.
5. Also pat along the child's entire spine for thirty minutes.
6. Slap the top and back of the head.
7. Next, slap the neck, shoulders, and the back of the hands.
8. In more severe cases, slap along the entire spine and the Urinary Bladder Meridian on both sides.
9. You can use a hair dryer to warm up the regions before *Paida*, particularly the neck and *Dazhui* Acupoints.
10. To relieve more severe symptoms, *Paida* longer and for additional rounds.
11. Drink ginger and jujube tea and do warm-water footbaths.
12. Stretch on a *Lajin* bench.
13. Do wall-hitting exercises or meditative jogging for over half an hour.

CONSTIPATION AND HEMORRHOIDS

1. Slap the back of the hands and the entire buttocks.
2. It's positive if colorful patches of *sha* appear.
3. For more severe symptoms, slap for multiple rounds until *sha* comes out and there is bleeding. This might be necessary.

CRAMPING

Slap on the inner elbows, the back of the feet, and around the impacted areas.

CRITICAL DISEASES

This category includes some so-called incurable diseases, such as:

- AIDS
- Myasthenia Gravis
- Parkinson's Disease
- Alzheimer's Disease
- Rheumatoid arthritis
- Ankylosing spondylitis (AS)
- Lupus erythematodes (LE)
- Osteonecrosis of the femoral head (ONFH)
- Tobacco, drug, and alcohol addiction

In Western Medicine, these diseases are disorders of almost all bodily systems including the immune, nervous, and digestive systems. According to Traditional Chinese Medicine, they are simply meridian blockages. Like in all cases, unblocking the meridians leads to healing—but it will take longer.

There can be visible improvements after one month. Many patients stop medication after practicing *PaidaLajin* and experience continual improvements. There are many testimonials of people improving or self-healing Alzheimer's disease and ONFH.

1. Stretch on a *Lajin* bench.
2. Slap the universal regions (elbows, knees, hands, and feet.)
3. Follow with the entire head, all four limbs, and all joints and regions of the body.
4. Include the chest, back, belly, groin, armpits, and buttocks.
5. During the process of *PaidaLajin* for chronic diseases, it is best to fast for three to four days.
6. People with weak *qi* and blood supply can also try fasting.

7. Drink some ginger and jujube tea to replenish *qi* and blood flow in the meantime.

It should be noted that prolonged medication, particularly hormonal drugs, are very harmful to a patient's health. They can lead to drug-induced and other iatrogenic diseases. You should consult with your doctor about reducing the dosage or stopping medication. Many patients have experienced better healing effects by practicing *PaidaLajin* after reducing the dosage or stopping medication.

Most of the patients with rare and critical diseases have undergone various treatments for years, but to no avail. Many have lost hope. They tend to be more vulnerable and afraid of pain. They need patient guidance and encouragement. *PaidaLajin* should be gradually implemented.

DIARRHEA AND FOOD POISONING

1. Slap the *Hegu* Acupoints, *Zusanli* Acupoints, *Neiguan* Acupoints, the back of the hands, and the abdomen.
2. Drink ginger and jujube tea.
3. Stretch on a *Lajin* bench.

DIABETES AND HYPERTENSION

Often patients suffer from diabetes, hypertension, and heart disease at the same time. It's one of the most typical groups of complex diseases. It's easy to be misled by the names of the diseases, heart rate, blood glucose measurements, and blood pressure levels.

It's simpler to break it down to the root cause: Heart disease.

These are also Heart diseases:

- Tumors
- Insomnia
- Depression

- Skin Disorders
- Mental Illness
- Liver and Kidney Problems
- Immune, Nervous, Digestive, and Respiratory System Disorders

Chinese Medicine concludes these are all cured through heart-felt change. When the Heart (the King of Bodily Organs) has problems, other internal organs (the government and military officials serving the king) take some of the burden, causing diseases in these organs. Healing the Heart takes the pressure off of the other systems.

In March 2015, we held a five-day clinical workshop in partnership with the TAG-VHS Diabetes Research Centre in Chennai, India. Most of the diabetic patients in attendance also had heart disease and hyper or hypotension.

Hyper and hypotension are connected to the Heart. You want to clean the Heart Meridian and Pericardium Meridians first. Blood will flow more naturally, and the body will produce various beneficial hormones. Conscientious *Paida* on the universal regions stimulates even more hormones, creating internal medicine.

Workshop participants voluntarily reduced their dosage of insulin or stopped it completely. (Note: please seek the approval of your doctor when making any changes to your medication.) They drank ginger and jujube tea with brown sugar in it. At the end of the workshop, their blood glucose and blood pressure levels naturally leveled out. Some patients continued *PaidaLajin* at home. Their levels continue to remain normal.

The fact diabetes was healed with only *PaidaLajin* proves diabetes isn't only connected to sugar intake. The body can't produce enough of its own insulin to regulate blood glucose.

Please refer the preliminary report on *PaidaLajin's* Clinical Research Workshop.

It's best to attend a *PaidaLajin* self-healing workshop to address these three chronic illnesses. If you practice at home and you're not strong enough to keep slapping and stretching two or three times a day. Try to at least *Paida*:

The Universal Regions:

- Elbows
- Knees
- Hands
- Feet

Follow with:

- Limbs
- Armpits
- Belly
- Groin

If possible, carpet bomb your entire body.

After health is balanced, focus more on the universal regions.

1. Slap all over the feet, including the sole, instep, inner and outer sides of the ankle, and the toes. Use a *Paida* stick if necessary. Slap each region for five to sixty minutes. To relieve more severe symptoms, *Paida* longer and for additional rounds.
2. After *sha* disappears, start a new round.
3. Drink ginger and jujube tea daily.
4. Use *PaidaLajin* to maintain good health.
5. Gradually lower the frequency and intensity.
6. Focus on the universal regions and the head.
7. Stretch regularly.
8. Make *PaidaLajin* an integral part of your daily life.

DIZZINESS WITH CRAMPS

In addition to the inner elbows and *Neiguan* Acupoints, slap the top of the feet.

NOTE: If someone is dizzy or in a coma, always treat it as an acute heart attack. Start with soft *Paida* and gradually increase the intensity.

EAR, NOSE, AND THROAT

1. Begin with *Lajin.*
2. *Paida* the universal regions (elbows, knees, hands, and feet.)
3. Slap along all four limbs to clear blockages that correspond to internal organs.
4. Then slap the entire head and face, especially the sick facial organ. The meridians on the head and face are closely related, and they form a network.

CAUTION: it is NOT advisable for people suffering from—or with the potential risk—of retinal detachment.

1. Cover each eye with an entire palm and slap. You are slapping the eye socket and not the eye itself.
2. For rhinitis, slap more on the forehead, cheeks, and inner elbows.
3. Slapping along meridians that correspond to these organs is very effective in healing these diseases.
4. Reference the previous correlations. For instance, *Paida* along the Kidney Meridian improves tinnitus and deafness, and *Paida* on the Liver Meridian with *Lajin* helps relieve eye problems.
5. You can find the corresponding meridians by referring to a meridians chart or just slap the universal regions (elbows,

knees, hands, and feet), since they cover all of the necessary meridians.

6. Slap each region for five to sixty minutes.
7. Practice Neck *Lajin* for five to sixty minutes.

EDEMA

To relieve edema, stretch on a *Lajin* bench, *Paida* the universal regions (elbows, knees, hands, and feet), and then slap all along the four limbs. The edema will disappear.

EMERGENCIES

Paida: Slap one region or acupoint for five to thirty minutes, depending on the severity of the problem (see pictures.) An even longer practice might be necessary in extreme cases.

Lajin: Like *Paida*, stretch one leg for five to thirty minutes, depending on the severity of the problem (see pictures.) Once again, you may need to extend the time in some instances.

- Emergencies
- Acute Heart Problems
- Unconsciousness
- Asthma Attacks
- Chest Tightness
- Shortness of Breath
- Nausea
- Vomiting
- Headaches
- Dizziness
- Alcohol poisoning
- Heat Stroke
- Motion Sickness
- Altitude Sickness

- Abnormal Sweating
- Uncontrollable shaking
- Purplish-Black Lips
- Pale or Greenish-Black Face
- Emotional Overreactions (Such as Joy, Rage, Anxiety, Agitation, or Depression)

1. Heavily slap inner elbows and the *Neiguan* Acupoints near the wrist.
2. If two people are available, each can take one arm. Otherwise, one person should slap both elbows and *Neiguan* Acupoints at the same time.
3. Then slap the entire inner side of each arm.
4. In severe cases, slap between the breasts and the corresponding area along the spine.

In an emergency, you may immediately use heavy slaps.

ENDOCRINE DISORDERS (SEE CHRONIC DISEASES)

GYNECOLOGICAL DISORDERS

Gynecological disorders are mostly cold-induced diseases connected to the heart, liver, spleen, and kidneys.

Women with gynecological disorders usually suffer depression, including postnatal depression. The severity of depression corresponds to the severity of the disorders. The fundamental cause of depression is problems with the Heart, including negative feelings such as fear, grief, anger, hatred, or jealousy.

Common disease names include:

- Annexitis
- Infertility
- Adenomyosis

- Ovarian cysts
- Uterine fibroids
- Breast hyperplasia
- Prolapsed uterus
- Irregular menstruation
- Menstrual pain

They are often accompanied by:

- Insomnia
- Depression
- Constipation
- Hair loss
- Hypothyroidism
- Hyperthyroidism

Often, women have several diseases simultaneously, such as hyperthyroidism, breast tumors, and uterine fibroids.

PaidaLajin for Gynecological Disorders

1. Stretch on a *Lajin* bench.
2. Slap the universal regions (elbows, knees, hands, and feet.)
3. *Paida* all four limbs and the Baliao Area (the upper middle buttocks, also called the sacrum.)
4. Cover the entire head, breasts, armpits, belly, buttocks, inner thighs, and groin.
5. Slap all over the body if you have time.
6. Slap each region for five to sixty minutes.
7. To relieve more severe symptoms, *Paida* longer and for additional rounds.
8. Drink ginger and jujube tea.
9. Do daily warm-water footbaths in 104° F water (40° C).

Breasts

Paida on the breasts is beneficial in many ways. All nine major meridians and body systems are closely related to the breasts. It helps diagnose and heal:

- Mammary gland diseases
- Problems with the uterus and ovaries
- Immune and digestive disorders
- Cardiovascular and cerebrovascular diseases

Vaginal Itchiness

Slap on the area (perineum), the groin, the belly, and the inner thighs.

Menstrual Pain

1. Do *Lajin* in Reclining, Squatting, or Y-Shaped Posture for twenty to thirty minutes.
2. Slap along the groin, the belly, and the inner sides of thighs and knees.
3. Slap each region for five to sixty minutes.
4. To relieve more severe symptoms, *Paida* longer and for additional rounds.
5. Practice wall hitting.
6. Drink ginger and jujube tea to enhance the circulation of *qi* and blood.
7. Stay warm.

HAND CRAMPS

1. Slap on *Neiguan* Acupoints, inner elbows, and both sides of the hands.

HEADACHES

1. Slap the painful spots on the head.
2. Follow with the rest of the head, the back of the hands, inner elbows, and the *Neiguan* Acupoints.
3. Move to the entire head, neck, shoulders, inner elbows, and back of hands.
4. Stretch on a *Lajin* bench.

HEALING REACTIONS

Whatever healing reactions occur, your top priority is to protect your heart.

According to Chinese Medicine, Heart is the king—in charge of everything pertaining to our wellbeing.

Common healing reactions include:

- Pain
- Chills
- Cramps
- Hunger
- Fatigue
- Nausea
- Vomiting
- Dizziness
- Insomnia
- Itchiness

The first step is to slap on the inner elbows and *Neiguan* Acupoints. The Heart, Pericardium, and Lung Meridians run through these areas, as well as other important acupoints.

In severe cases, slap heavily. Then slap all along the inner side of each arm. If someone is in a coma, two people can simultaneously slap on the patient's inner elbows and *Neiguan* Acupoints on both arms.

HEART DISEASE

***Paida* the Heart and Pericardium Meridians in the inner elbows to prove heart disease.**

Almost everyone will have *sha* and feel pain. It shows almost everyone has heart disease, though the severity varies.

Sudden heart attacks occur when the Heart is extremely blocked. A person dies when their heart is completely blocked. In theory, we know the importance of disease prevention. However, most people still wait until they have a heart attack or another severe illness—related to the Heart—before they seek treatment.

They don't want to practice *PaidaLajin* now, because it hurts. They don't want to attend a *PaidaLajin* workshop, because they feel they don't have time for it. However, when they have a stroke or a heart attack, they are compelled to go to the hospital.

Why does the Heart get sick so easily?

Because it is hurt the most deeply and frequently.

Beginning in childhood, we are faced with pressure concerning studying, love, work, family, and other relationships. Negative energy and emotions arise and are accumulated in the body, including fear, worry, stress, anger, hatred, sorrow, and jealousy. All these negative feelings hurt the Heart directly, leading to a tightening of the Heart—just like a cold-induced contraction. This, in turn, leads to the contraction of tendons and ligaments all over the body. That is how we get sick.

In other words, stress and negative emotions lead to contraction and obstruction of the Heart Meridian, which results in blockages in other meridians and internal organs.

Before all else, the Heart and Pericardium Meridians should be cleared of blockages. We always recommend slapping the inner elbows and *Neiguan* Acupoints first, for they are very closely linked to the heart. To relieve more severe symptoms, you can also *Paida* the chest and back, particularly the area in between the breasts and the corresponding area on the back.

Patients with heart disease tend to be more afraid of pain than others. The more severe the heart disease is, the more afraid of pain the patients are. This is because the Heart feels the pain and discomfort from all parts of the body. There is a saying, "The fingers are linked to the Heart." Indeed, when the fingers are injured, it is the Heart that feels the pain.

There are two types of cardiac patients: those with excessive qi and those with weak *qi*.

Excessive *Qi*

Generally:

- Hypertensive
- Often male
- Overweight
- Sweat heavily
- Dislike heat
- Love cold drinks and air-conditioning

They appear to feel hot externally, but deep inside their heart is freezing cold. The deficient kidney functions can't keep the *yang* inside the body, and heat leaks out as they constantly sweat. They may appear to be alright, but they face the dangers of sudden heart attacks and strokes. They may also suffer from:

- Dizziness
- Headaches
- Diabetes
- Hypertension
- Impotence
- Premature ejaculation
- Prostate disorders

- Waist and knee pain
- Cancer

Weak *Qi*

Generally:

- Hypotensive
- Often female
- Overly thin
- Rarely sweat
- Love warmth
- Can't tolerate cold

Most suffer from:

- Insomnia
- Headaches
- Dizziness
- Infertility
- Depression
- Constipation
- Hypothyroidism
- Hyperthyroidism
- Hair loss
- Back pain
- Waist pain
- Menstrual pain and disorders
- Ovarian cysts
- Breast cancer
- Uterine fibroids
- Low blood sugar
- Low blood pressure
- Uterine prolapse
- Cold hands and feet

Whether excessive or deficient *qi*, hypertension or hypotension, they have a common problem with their Heart.

Heart disease can be felt as discomfort in the physical heart and other parts of the body. Fear, worry, anger, hatred, tension, jealousy, and other complex psychological entanglements—can they be detected with an instrument? A person becomes ill when they become too busy, both physically and psychologically, with family (especially children), career, their country, or other causes.

Many people feel palpitations, chest tightness, and other obvious symptoms indicating heart disease. However, when they go for a medical checkup, there are no findings. Sometimes, even when a patient with a heart attack is taken to the emergency room, the checkup does not show heart disease. It is said they "are in poor health."

Poor health can be more dangerous than known illnesses. When you wait until mild symptoms become diseases, symptoms become serious. The pain of *PaidaLajin* and *sha* are accurate indicators of potential health problems. When medication and surgery come into play, patients can further deteriorate. This leads to more medicine and operations, dragging people into a vicious cycle of life-long medication. Very often, patients die—not of the initial illness—but from drug-induced and other iatrogenic diseases developed during treatment.

Make a list of your worries and concerns. Decide if your loved ones and the world will cease to exist if you let go of your fears.

If you can really let go, much of your illness will be gone. If you can't:

1. *Paida* your inner elbows, limbs, chest, back, and entire body for five to thirty minutes per region.
2. Stretch on a *Lajin* bench for ten to thirty minutes per leg.
3. Be grateful and repent during *PaidaLajin*.

If this doesn't help:

1. Attend a *PaidaLajin* workshop.
2. Practice meditation.
3. Try meditative jogging, waist swirling, wall hitting, and *tie qiang gong* (see video tutorials on the English website.)
4. Self-heal your illnesses.

HYPERTENSION (SEE DIABETES AND HYPERTENSION)

ITCHINESS

1. Slap on the itchy areas, inner side of each knee, inner elbows, and the *Neiguan* Acupoints.
2. The efficacy is improved when the patient also stretches on a *Lajin* bench.
3. It is best to quickly and consume less food during this time. This allows *PaidaLajin* to burn wastes and toxins and turn them into treasured energy the body needs. Otherwise, the energy will be used to digest food, and you will see less results.
4. You can drink some ginger and jujube tea to nourish your *qi* and blood.

JOINT PAIN

Common joint pain includes neck pain, shoulder pain, wrist pain, hand pain, lower back pain, leg pain, and ankle pain.

1. In all cases, slap directly on the connected areas for fifteen minutes to an hour.
2. *Paida* longer and for additional rounds for more severe pain.
3. Always start with soft *Paida* and gradually slap harder.

Neck Pain

1. Slap the entire neck and the shoulders.
2. Stretch on a *Lajin* bench.
3. Another option: practice the wall-hitting exercise.
4. Neck pain and headaches during both are normal.

Frozen Shoulders

1. Slap the front, back, left, right, upper, and lower parts of the shoulders.
2. Slap the armpits.
3. Stretch on a *Lajin* bench and do *Lajin* in Standing Posture.
4. Take turns doing *Paida* and *Lajin*.

Lower Back and Leg Pain

1. Stretch on a *Lajin* bench.
2. Slap on the painful areas and all around the knees.
3. For severe pain, *Paida* all around the legs.
4. Take turns doing *Paida* and *Lajin*.

Wrist and Ankle Pain

1. Slap the upper and lower parts of the painful areas and all around them.
2. Drink ginger and jujube tea to enhance the circulation of *qi* and blood.

KIDNEY DEFICIENCY

Deficient Kidney *yang* leads to cold limbs and fear of the cold.

Deficient Kidney *yin* leads to fear of heat, hot palms and feet, and low fevers and night sweats.

Paida is the best way to boost *yang*.

1. Focus on the universal regions and the entire spine.
2. Then *Paida* the head, chest, belly, back, and buttocks.
3. Move on to carpet bomb the entire body.
4. *Lajin* in Reclining Posture, in addition to the Urinary Bladder Meridian, also stretches the Liver, Spleen, and Kidney Meridians. The Liver Meridian goes directly through the male genitalia.
5. Reclining Posture also stretches the Lung, Heart, Pericardium, and Big and Small Intestine Meridians. Strong hearts and lungs are important for both nourishment and sexuality.

Additional *Paida* to Energize the Kidneys

Paida the head and face to boost the entire body.

Six *yang* meridians go up to the head, and the health of all internal organs is reflected on the face. We recommend this sequence:

- Top of the head
- Left and right sides of the head
- Front and back sides of the head
- Neck
- Eye sockets
- Cheeks
- Mouth
- Ears

The Stomach Meridian goes through the cheeks.
The Spleen Meridian goes through the mouth.
The Lung Meridian goes through the nose.
The Kidney Meridian goes through the ears.
The Liver Meridian goes through the eyes.

The Gall Bladder Meridian goes along the left and right sides of the head.
The Urinary Bladder Meridian goes along the front and back sides of the head and neck.

While patting eye sockets and cheeks, the nose is also stimulated. You can slap all these parts or choose to focus on certain areas. In our workshop, the participants spend over an hour on these each morning.

KIDNEY FAILURE, NEPHRITIS, AND DIALYSIS

These illnesses are common among men and women, young and old. For a large number of patients, they are caused by medication for other illnesses. In this case, all internal organs have severe problems, particularly the heart, liver, spleen, and kidneys.

The treatments for these diseases are long and alarmingly expensive. Kidney dialysis in particular can be a huge financial burden on individuals, families, and governments.

However, these diseases can be improved and self-healed with *PaidaLajin*. The key is changing the mindset of the patient.

The following meridians are blocked:

- Heart
- Liver
- Spleen
- Kidney
- Stomach
- Gall Bladder
- Urinary Bladder
- Big and Small Intestine

1. Slap the universal regions (elbows, knees, hands and feet) first.
2. Slap along the four limbs.

3. Slap the hands and feet for a long time.
4. Carpet bomb the entire body.
5. Slap each region for five to sixty minutes each time.
6. To relieve more severe symptoms, *Paida* longer and for additional rounds.
7. When *sha* disappears, start a new round of *Paida*.
8. Do several rounds of carpet bombing.
9. Stretch one to three times a day for five to forty minutes per leg each time.
10. Add sandbags weighing eleven pounds to each leg.
11. Drink ginger and jujube daily.

There have been records of both children and adults successfully self-healing kidney failure. During the process of *PaidaLajin*, the patient can experience pain, nausea, vomiting, diarrhea, dizziness, and fainting. These are good signs.

Slap on the inner elbows and *Neiguan* Acupoints to relieve healing reactions. Rest well and continue *PaidaLajin*. DO NOT stop *PaidaLajin* because of any of the healing reactions. DO NOT view the reward as a punishment.

LEG AND FEET CRAMPS

1. Slap the inner elbows, tops of feet, all around the knees, and the entire calves.

LIVER AND GALL BLADDER PAIN

1. Slap the inner and outer sides of both legs.
2. Stretch on a *Lajin* bench or stand on a *Lajin* standing board.
3. Slap the *Neiguan* Acupoints and the inner elbows.

LUPUS (SEE CRITICAL DISEASES)

MENTAL DISORDERS, INCLUDING DEPRESSION

The body, mind, and soul are one. They interact with and impact one another. Patients with depression or other mental disorders suffer from many physical illnesses as well. In fact, all the internal organs are malfunctioning, particularly the heart, liver, spleen, kidneys, and intestines. Their corresponding meridians and the brain are very clogged.

1. *Paida* the universal regions (elbows, knees, hands, and feet) first.
2. Slap along the four limbs.
3. Slap the entire head, chest, back, armpits, and groin.
4. Focus more on inner elbows, *Neiguan* Acupoints, head, hands, and feet.
5. Slap each region for five to sixty minutes each time.
6. To relieve more severe symptoms, *Paida* longer and for additional rounds.
7. A patient with severe depression has even more severe heart problems.
8. Inner elbow skin might break, causing toxic blood and fluid to seep out. The patient will recover faster.
9. A patient with depression tends to cry during *Paida*. Involuntary crying is a good healing reaction that clears toxins from the heart. It also helps open the Heart.
10. Leave the patient to cry it all out.
11. After the crying, slapping and stretching can continue.
12. Stretch one to three times a day.
13. Drink ginger and jujube tea daily.

MYASTHENIA GRAVIS (SEE CRITICAL DISEASES)

NEUROLOGICAL DISORDERS (SEE CHRONIC DISEASES)

NOSE BLEEDS

Slap the inner elbows and the back of both hands.

ORGAN PAIN

Common organ pain includes:

- Headaches
- Toothaches
- Abdominal pain
- Stomachaches
- Liver pain
- Gall bladder pain
- Menstrual pain

Slap the major regions along relevant meridians by referring to a meridians chart. Since most people are unfamiliar with meridians and acupoints, it is easier to slap body parts. Each covers multiple meridians and acupoints.

OSTEONECROSIS OF THE FEMORAL HEAD (ONFH)

1. Follow steps for critical illnesses.
2. Focus more on stretching on a *Lajin* bench.
3. Do waist swirling: swirl in a horizontal circle to boost kidney energy, like doing a hoola hoop. (See the video tutorial on our English website.)
4. *Tie qiang gong*: stand with your nose close to wall, squat down, and then stand up. (See video tutorial on the English website.)

5. Slap the impacted areas for five to sixty minutes.
6. To relieve more severe symptoms, *Paida* longer and for additional rounds.

PARKINSON'S DISEASE (SEE CRITICAL DISEASES)

PEDIATRIC DISEASES

Children mainly suffer from such digestive and respiratory problems as colds, fevers, eczema, coughing, vomiting, or diarrhea.

Children Under a Year Old

1. Pat along the entire spine for over half an hour.
2. To relieve more severe symptoms, pat the universal regions (elbows, knees, hands, and feet.)
3. Pat the *Zusanli* Acupoints and all four limbs.
4. Pat each region for fifteen minutes to an hour.
5. To relieve more severe symptoms, *Paida* longer and for additional rounds.

Children Over a Year Old

1. Follow the above steps and include stretching on a *Lajin* bench.
2. Parents who know chiropractic massage can use it alternately with *Paida*.
3. *Paida* provides greater stimulation to the internal organs than massage. You can take turns between the two.
4. Use a hair dryer to blow warm air at a child's illness-related regions until the skin gets red and hot. It helps *qi* and blood flow more smoothly.

Children typically respond more to *Paida* because their diseases are usually simpler. They also generally have enough *yang*. Children don't generally suffer from as many psychological disorders as adults. They don't judge *Paida*, and they accept it with an open mind.

Pat softly most of the time. Intense *Paida* is not the key to healing pediatric diseases. What matters more is the Heart—love, focus, and confidence. Some parents don't notice an improvement after patting their children. This is usually because the adult is anxious or tired. They don't put enough positive energy into the practice.

A child may be frightened the first time you blow warm air at him or her. Stay calm and guide the child to love the "toy." Blow the hair dryer at yourself and make faces. Gradually, your child will get used to it. If you have any concerns, use a warm water bag instead.

Paida and Massage for Common Pediatric Diseases

- Colds
- Fever
- Coughing
- Constipation
- Indigestion
- Pneumonia
- Sore Throat
- Runny Nose
- Pediatric Asthma
- Spitting Up Milk
- Inexplicable Crying
- Restlessness

If the symptoms aren't severe, gently pat the child's *Dazhui* Acupoints. Then use a hair dryer to warm up *Dazhui* Acupoints and the entire body. It is best to see *sha* or red and hot skin.

Fever, Coughing, and More Severe Symptoms

1. Gently pat the child's *Dazhui* Acupoints and their entire spine.

2. Use chiropractic manipulation along the child's spine.
3. Warm up the child's body with a hair dryer or a warm water bag.
4. It is best to see *sha* or red and hot skin.

Even More Severe Symptoms

1. Pat the child's universal regions (elbows, knees, hands, and feet.)
2. Pat their chest and back.
3. Sometimes, their fever might return a second or third time.
4. Stay calm and repeat the above actions.
5. *Paida Yongquan* Acupoints.

Rashes, Eczema, and Other Skin Allergies

1. Directly pat the itchy or damaged areas.
2. Warm up those areas and the entire spine.
3. It is best to see *sha* or red and hot skin.
4. If their condition doesn't improve, also pat the universal regions (elbows, knees, hands, and feet.)

KEEPING YOUR CHILD HEALTHY

Pat and massage their entire spine, *Zusanli* Acupoints, and *Yongquan* Acupoints once or twice a day. Massage each acupoint or pat an area for several minutes.

Please Note:

1. Sometimes children have recurring fevers.
2. When the child's forehead is hot while their ears are cool, it is not a disease. It's a physiological response. After the fever is gone, the child's health will improve.

3. Several *Paida* and massage sessions may be needed.
4. Many pediatric diseases are caused by excessive eating and drinking, or too many clothes on a child.
5. We recommend less food intake or fasting when a child is sick in any way.
6. Don't force children to eat and drink more.
7. During *PaidaLajin*, fever and coughing often relapse. These are normal healing reactions. Continue with *PaidaLajin*. For cold-induced colds and fevers, drink some ginger and jujube tea.

PREGNANCY AND CHILDBIRTH

Initially, we discouraged pregnant women from practicing *PaidaLajin* as a matter of caution. However, many pregnant women began practicing it on their own. The results show that *PaidaLajin* not only helps heal common pregnancy distresses without the need for medication—it also facilitates natural delivery of babies. Moreover, it is beneficial to the growth of the baby before and after birth.

PaidaLajin in pregnant women addresses:

- Pain
- Edema
- Insomnia
- Nausea
- Vomiting
- Diarrhea
- Constipation
- Skin disorders
- Heart disease
- Kidney disease

CAUTION:

Pregnant women should avoid slapping their belly. It is OK to slap other parts of the body and stretch on a *Lajin* bench.

The women who benefit the most from *PaidaLajin* are those who practice it every day during pregnancy for health preservation. The recommended *PaidaLajin* regimes for healing various diseases are applicable to pregnant women as well.

1. Slap the universal regions (elbows, knees, hands, and feet.)
2. *Paida* the head.
3. Move on to the four limbs.
4. The intensity and frequency of *Paida* can be adjusted.
5. Slap each region for five to sixty minutes each time.
6. To relieve more severe symptoms, *Paida* longer and for additional rounds.

Natural Childbirth

PaidaLajin is very helpful for natural delivery. Some pregnant women who persisted in *PaidaLajin* completed natural delivery of their baby in half an hour, without the need for a Cesarean section. *PaidaLajin* makes the muscles, tendons, and ligaments of the hip-bones and birth canal more flexible. More importantly, the Liver, Spleen, and Kidney Meridians linked to the womb and birth canal are cleared of blockages, thus facilitating the delivery.

PaidaLajin is even more essential for a woman after childbirth. It assists with:

- Pain
- Fevers
- Obesity
- Mastitis
- Insomnia

- Postpartum depression
- Uneven milk supply

1. *Paida* the universal regions (elbows, knees, hands, and feet.)
2. Move to the breasts, belly, and the Baliao Area (the upper middle buttocks, also called the sacrum.)

After childbirth, practice *Lajin* more often. *Paida* and *Lajin* combined help a woman recover her muscle structure after childbirth. It facilitates a normal milk supply and helps with infant care. Women who persist in postnatal *PaidaLajin* can expect to return to their normal health condition within a month.

PROSTATE AND URINARY DISORDERS

Prostate disorders are quite common among elderly men.

Over 90% of men over seventy years old suffer from such problems as prostatitis, prostate enlargement, and prostate cancer. Common symptoms include urgent, frequent, and incomplete urination, and local pain and swelling. Many women, after childbirth, suffer from urethritis, frequent urination, and urinary incontinence. Urinary disorders in both men and women lead to frequent bathroom visits at night.

The Kidney and Urinary Bladder Meridians regulate water channels in the body. All internal organs are related to these disorders.

1. Follow our recommendations for kidney deficiency.
2. Focus more on slapping the inner side of each thigh, groin, lower abdomen, and buttocks.
3. When the condition improves, gradually slap along the limbs and feet to thoroughly detoxify.
4. Slap each region for five to sixty minutes each time.
5. To relieve more severe symptoms, *Paida* longer and for additional rounds.

6. Stretch one to three times a day.
7. Gradually extend the duration up to thirty minutes per leg each time.
8. Add sandbags weighing 6.5–33 pounds to each leg.

We have countless records and testimonials of patients with prostate disorders who have self-healed with *PaidaLajin*. The most dramatic case is an eighty-six-year-old patient with terminal prostate cancer. His cancer was cured thanks to his daughter's high-powered *Paida* over a period of almost three months. Sometimes, she would slap one of his legs for four and a half hours. The patient yelled the entire time, but the "torture" cured his cancer and other illnesses as well. Chemotherapy is torture because you're poisoning your body, and we have found it to be less effective than *PaidaLajin*.

Please visit our website to learn more about healing miracles.

RHEUMATOID ARTHRITIS (SEE CRITICAL DISEASES)

SCOLIOSIS

Scoliosis is a back problem that causes the spine to curve to one side. It forces a person to hunch over. Persistent *PaidaLajin* returns the bones to their proper position, makes the tendons flexible, improves *qi* and blood circulation, and increases the height of the patient. It has proven effective in men and women, young and old. Some old people become taller because *PaidaLajin* causes intervertebral distances to increase.

Almost all workshop participants have experienced these by-products of self-healing.

It is not unusual for someone to lose eleven to forty-five pounds in one to six months.

SENSORY ORGAN DISORDERS

- Eyes
- Ears
- Noses
- Mouths
- Teeth
- Tongues

Issues with the sensory organs are superficial symptoms. The root causes are their respective internal organs.

According to Chinese Medicine:

- **Eye** problems relate to the **liver.**
- **Ear** and **tooth** problems relate to the **kidneys.**
- **Nose** problems relate to the **lungs.**
- **Lip, cheek,** and other **facial muscle** problems relate to the **spleen.**
- **Tongue** problems relate to the **heart.**

SEXUAL DISORDERS

Over the past few years, I have received countless emails inquiring whether *PaidaLajin* can improve sexual dysfunction. This problem not only applies to personal health—but can also impact the harmony within a family.

According to Chinese health statistics, the incidence of illness and medication-induced erectile dysfunction (ED) in adult males is at least 10%. This figure does not include those who avoid seeking medical treatment. Erectile dysfunction can be either organic or psychological. But the essence is the same—a functional disorder is a complex disease caused by blockages in a number of meridians.

Sexual dysfunction in men and women can have different origins: A man is mostly concerned about the size and function of his penis, particularly the potential problems of impotence and premature ejaculation. In fact, the size and strength of his penis are superficial manifestations of the more crucial "software" driving it, enough smoothly flowing *qi*. By contrast, a woman's sexual dysfunction can often result from concerns about the visual beauty of her figure, particularly the size and shape of her breasts and buttocks, and the smoothness of her skin.

Despite their different concerns, men and women's sexual disorders are fundamentally the same problem with *qi*. Enough *qi* brings fullness, function, and beauty. Insufficient *qi* results in atrophy, dysfunction, and a lack of beauty. In short, *qi* is vital to sexuality.

Imagine a man's penis is like a balloon. With enough *qi*, it inflates; without enough *qi* or *qi* leakage, it shrinks. An overweight man tends to suffer kidney deficiency and shortness of breath. His body may look big, while his penis is tiny. When I was a child, I used to go to a public bathhouse. We boys used to comment on adult men's penises, and we discovered a surprise finding: Normally, an obese man's penis looked like an almost invisible screw. We wondered why a big man should have a smaller penis. When I became an adult myself, I found that some men have a large, but soft, unsustainable penis. Later on, I learned that these all resulted from the same problems.

Qi also determines whether a woman's breasts look beautiful in size and shape. A woman's skin will dry out and her breasts will shrink as she ages because her *yang* weakens. In fact, a woman's sexual dysfunction manifests as various diseases and symptoms:

- Anger
- Fatigue
- Insomnia
- Depression
- Constipation

- Waist pain
- *Qi* deficiency
- Irregular heartbeat
- Gynecological disorders
- Hot upper body
- Cold lower limbs
- An irritating hot sensation in the palms, soles of the feet, and the chest

Many of these symptoms appear during menopause; however, some women have such symptoms at around forty. It's called early menopause syndrome or perimenopause.

Of course, *qi* here does not refer to the air, but the level of *yang* in a person. Chinese people often say, "*Qi* sustains a person's life." In the phrases "good *qi* color in the face," and "lose all the dead *qi*", *qi* refers to *yang*. According to Chinese Medicine, *qi* propels blood flow. That is to say, it is *qi* that moves blood along the vessels. Although a man's penis—and a woman's breasts and vagina—have inflatable tissues, it is *qi* that determines their functioning—not blood or nerve cells. In short, where there is sexual apathy or dysfunction, there is deficient *yang*.

Then comes the next question: How to boost *yang*? Take nourishing foods and supplements? Haven't there been enough such drugs and supplements from ancient times till today? Consider the dog penis, Chinese pilose antler, Viagra, and other Western biochemical drugs. Don't they deplete a man's *yang*, have negative effects, and even make him die earlier? If drugs and supplements really work, kings and the richest men in human history should've been the healthiest and lived the longest. But it has never been so.

Taking drugs, hormones, and other supplements often damages internal organs and leads to many drug-induced diseases. Read the drug instructions carefully, and you will find that drugs for insomnia, diabetes, depression, hypertension, heart disease, and other common illnesses have a number of negative effects that damage internal organs, impair *yang*, and block meridians. Some people take drugs to control blood glucose and blood pressure levels, but they suffer weakening liver, spleen, and kidney functions. They experience poor or no sexuality.

Natural *yang* connects with the energy of the universe. Energy is a vibration frequency that regulates the boundless universe and all forms of life in a subtle and accurate way. The meridian system in the human body provides channels for energy flow. Smooth energy flow in meridians equals great nourishment. The heart, liver, kidneys, urinary bladder, and their corresponding meridians are involved in the process of balancing sufficient amounts of *yang*.

Many Chinese people believe renal function determines sexual function. In fact, the heart—King of Organs—is the most crucial. When the Heart is not at peace, the entire kingdom (the human body) will be a mess. Our desires and aspirations originate from the Heart, and it's the seat of a person's vitality. Without the power of the Heart, a person has no desires at all, including sexual desire. They may already be depressed.

In men: impotence, a soft penis, spermatorrhea, premature ejaculation, and infertility

In women: constipation, menstrual disorders, poor uterine growth, decreased sexual desire, and infertility

In both men and women:

- Premature aging
- Alzheimer's symptoms
- Backaches
- Osteoporosis
- Forgetfulness
- Leg pain

- Hair loss
- Hearing loss
- Loose teeth
- Poor eyesight
- Premature gray hair.
- Excretory dysfunction
- Edema
- Constipation
- Urgent, frequent, and incomplete urination
- Constipation might cause anal fissure and hemorrhoids

The Liver, Spleen and Kidney Meridians run along the inner side of each leg.

The Urinary Bladder Meridian moves along the back of each leg.

The Heart and Pericardium Meridians are along the inner side of each arm.

Lajin clears the Liver Meridian, giving the penis energy.

1. *Paida* the universal regions (elbows, knees, hands, and feet.)
2. Focus on the Heart, Kidney, Liver, and Urinary Bladder Meridians.
3. Slap all four limbs, particularly the armpits, groin, and the inner side of each leg. The Eight Weak Corners (armpits, groin, inner elbows, and back of the knees) along the limbs are most closely linked to sexual organs.
4. Carpet bomb the entire body.
5. Slap each region at a moderate pain intensity for five to sixty minutes.
6. To relieve more severe symptoms, *Paida* longer and for additional rounds.

SKIN DISEASES

Skin diseases exhibit internal organ problems that manifest on the skin. These include:

- Skin pain
- Sores
- Ulcers
- Allergies
- Itchiness
- Dryness

All are the results of toxins being excreted from internal organs. The *Huang Di Nei Jing* clearly states, "All pain, sores, and itchiness originate from the Heart."

Hives, Eczema, Psoriasis, Mosquito and Other Insect Bites, and Itchiness

1. Slap the itchy and damaged areas.
2. Move on to the universal regions (elbows, knees, hands, and feet.)
3. *Paida* the inner thighs.
4. Drink ginger and jujube tea.
5. Stretch on a *Lajin* bench.

Rashes, Itchiness, and Bites from Insects or Toxic Animals

1. Directly slap the bitten area. Blood and toxic fluid should come out of the skin.
2. Use a *Paida* tool for hard-to-reach body parts.

For areas that are very itchy, heavily slap extremely itchy areas until you see colorful patches of *sha*, reddish swelling. The skin might break, and fluid might seep out.

Dermatitis, Neurodermatitis, Allergic Contact Dermatitis (ACD), and Hard Skin

Treat these as problems with internal organs, particularly the heart, liver, spleen, lungs, and kidneys.

1. Slap the universal regions (elbows, knees, hands, and feet.)
2. Move to the damaged areas.
3. Slap the entire body, emphasizing the four limbs.
4. If the skin breaks and blood and pus come out, continue slapping to clear it.
5. Slap each region for five to sixty minutes.
6. *Paida* longer and for additional rounds as needed.
7. Stretching on a *Lajin* bench, gradually extending it to sixty minutes per leg. Add a ten or twenty-two-pound sandbag to each leg if possible.
8. Drink ginger and jujube tea daily.

SKIN, WEIGHT, AND HEIGHT

People who persist in *PaidaLajin* can get taller and slimmer. In some cases, they might gain weight if they have been too thin. They become better looking because they are healthy. Obesity, acne, pimples, freckles, rough skin, and color spots are signs of health problems. Skin and weight problems are related to:

- Insomnia
- Diabetes
- Hypertension
- Depression
- Constipation
- Heart, kidney, spleen and stomach problems
- Gynecological disorders

1. Stretching on a *Lajin* bench can help tighten breasts. When lying on the *Lajin* bench with your arms stretching backward, your breasts are pulled upward, enhancing their elasticity.
2. Stretch first.
3. Focus on slapping the universal regions (elbows, knees, hands, and feet.)
4. Slap the breasts, belly, waist, buttocks, and thighs where a lot of fat and toxins tend to accumulate.
5. Slap cheeks for severe color spots.
6. Target other areas such as the limbs, hands, and feet.
7. Slap each region for five to sixty minutes each time.
8. To relieve more severe symptoms, *Paida* longer and for additional rounds.
9. The majority of overly thin people suffer from various chronic diseases, particularly spleen and stomach problems.
10. Focus more on slapping the universal regions (elbows, knees, hands, and feet), *Zusanli* Acupoints, and the four limbs.
11. Drink ginger and jujube tea.
12. Do daily warm-water footbaths in 104° F water (40° C).
13. With persistent *PaidaLajin* practice, it is natural to reach a healthy weight.

SORE THROAT AND TONSILS

Slap the front and sides of the neck, chest, back, hands, and feet.

SPLEEN AND STOMACH

The six meridians related to the spleen and stomach will be cleared: the Liver, Spleen, Stomach, Kidney, Gall Bladder, and Urinary Bladder Meridians.

1. Stretch on a *Lajin* bench one to two times a day.
2. *Paida* the universal regions (elbows, knees, hands and feet), the four limbs, and the belly.
3. *Paida* the *Zusanli* Acupoints along the Stomach Meridian regularly.
4. Do meditation and meditative standing, because excessive thinking hurts the spleen.
5. Zen jogging, wall hitting, waist swirling, and *tie qiang gong* exercises can also effectively improve spleen and stomach function.
6. Practice healthy eating that supports both nutrients and absorption. If the oil tube is blocked, you can't start the car—no matter how good the gasoline is.

STIFF FINGERS

1. Slap the back of the hands and the fingers.
2. Slap one hand for one to two hours until it swells up and *sha* thoroughly appears.
3. Slap the back of the other hand.
4. Slap the insteps of both feet for one to two hours, until they swell up and *sha* thoroughly appears.
5. Drink ginger and jujube tea.
6. Do daily warm-water footbaths in 104° F water (40° C).
7. Stretch one to three times per day.

STOMACHACHES AND NAUSEA

Slap on the *Zusanli* Acupoints, inner elbows, *Neiguan* Acupoints, and the back of the hands.

STROKES, INCLUDING PARALYSIS

1. Slap the inner elbows and the *Neiguan* Acupoints on each arm and both hands.
2. When the acute symptoms are gone, slap the universal regions (elbows, knees, hands, and feet), and then along the limbs.
3. Slap both sides of the body.
4. Then slap the entire head, including the top, left, right, front, and back sides.
5. Slap the neck and the cheeks.
6. If they have difficulty speaking, focus more on the head, cheeks, and the back of the hands.
7. Then carpet bomb all over the body.
8. Slap each region for five to sixty minutes each time.
9. To relieve more severe symptoms, *Paida* longer and for additional rounds.
10. Do daily warm-water footbaths in 104° F water (40° C).

Generally, these patients love to eat meat, eat too much or too often, and are very afraid of pain. Encourage them to eat less and go vegetarian. It's best to fast one day a week, or to always skip supper.

Paralyzed patients feel excruciating pain doing either *Paida* or *Lajin*. However, the more *PaidaLajin* they can do the better.

In 2011, when I visited Tibet for a second time, I met a lama (a guru) with stroke-induced paralysis who had been bedridden for three years. He was treated with four hours of intensive *PaidaLajin* by seven or eight young lamas. It was a very painful, and his two layers of clothes were soaked with sweat. After *PaidaLajin*, he was able to walk with crutches. The following day, he came again and received another four hours of *PaidaLajin*. Again, the young lamas slapped him. He howled in pain during the entire process. This time, he did not need the crutches at all anymore. He was able to walk slowly on his own feet.

In my experience, this was the fastest case of *PaidaLajin* healing stroke-induced paralysis.

TOOTHACHES

1. Slap the inner elbows and the back of the hands (particularly the *Hegu* Acupoints—between the thumb and index finger.)
2. You can also directly slap the cheeks and the mouth.

WAIST, BACK, AND LEG PAIN

1. Slap the back of the knees (including *Weizhong* Acupoints), and the back and outer sides of the legs.
2. You can also slap directly on the injured or painful areas.
3. Start soft and gradually go heavier.
4. Do *Lajin* in Reclining Posture.

17

RESEARCH, CLINICAL STUDIES, AND SURVERY RESULTS

HEALING REACTIONS, ACCORDING TO TRADITIONAL CHINESE MEDICINE (TCM)

Healing Crisis: A Sign of Recovery from a Major illness

This is an excerpt from an article by Mr. Liu Xiyan, a researcher of Traditional Chinese Medicine (TCM.)

"While curing a grave, chronic illness, a patient can often experience worse symptoms and discomforts after taking Chinese Medicine; in other words, he or she will experience healing crises before full recovery.

If you are very sick or have been sick for long, and have not experienced a healing crisis after taking much Chinese Medicine, then most likely your illness will not be cured, for you were not treated by a genuine TCM doctor; if you are a TCM doctor and have given countless prescriptions to your patients, but none of them have felt any healing reactions, then you will most likely think that Chinese Medicine indeed works slowly, for you are not a genuine TCM doctor.

The concept of healing crisis first appeared in the ancient Chinese classic *Shangshu* over two millennia ago. In the section "On Life" it says, 'A grave, chronic illness will not be cured if no healing crisis is felt after medication.' Later, Chinese texts explained that healing crises refer to discomforts felt during treatment.

In his book *Shang Han Lun* (also known as Discussion of Cold-Induced Disorders), Zhang Zhongjing, revered as Sage of Chinese Medicine, included several entries on healing crises.

For instance:

"After medication, the symptoms will be slightly relieved, and the patient will feel dizzy and restless. In severe cases, the nose will bleed. After nose-bleeding, the illness will be cured."

"After taking three prescriptions of Chinese Medicine, the patient will feel dizzy and listless. Do not panic. White atractylodes rhizome and monkshood are taking effect beneath the skin and haven't fully driven out dampness."

"After taking *chai hu tang*, the patient will tremble and then have warm sweats. After that comes recovery."

Dr. Hu Xishu (1898–1984, a renowned TCM doctor in contemporary China) repeatedly stressed that a patient could easily experience healing crises after taking *chai hu tang*. Specifically, the patient could shiver with chills and then sweat a lot.

Dr. Hu said, "If a practitioner is very healthy, there won't be healing reactions."

Dr. Hu cautioned doctors and patients to be aware of this healing cycle. He himself had been woken up at midnight because of a patient's healing crisis. The diarrhea patient was a child, and after drinking Dr. Hu's prescribed medicine, the diarrhea became even worse. His family members knocked on Dr. Hu's door at midnight, insisting he see the child. When Dr. Hu arrived there, the child's condition was already significantly improved.

Then Dr. Hu said, "Give the child the medicinal soup again."

Initially, the child's mother was afraid to do so. But after drinking the soup, the child fully recovered the next day.

In cases of healing crises, the doctor needs to stand firm and shouldn't acquiesce and change the prescription. Additionally, the doctor needs to explain clearly to the patient what is happening. All healing efforts will be wasted if the patient becomes frightened and goes for emergency treatment.

Healing crises are detox reactions or recovery responses during disease treatment. When the medicine is fighting off a disease, positive and negative energies in the body are engaged in a battle. Various discomforts can appear. When the positive energy is winning the battle, the negative energy will gradually recede. For patients with a grave, chronic illness, it is very likely for them to experience healing crises, which are signs of improvement leading to recovery.

Healing crises can last for several days. Some healing reactions are mild, and some are very severe. The forms and severity of healing crises vary from person to person. The sicker and weaker a patient is, and the longer the disease has been present, the more likely the patient is to experience strong healing reactions after taking the correct medicine.

In my clinical practice, I have encountered such healing crises as rashes, sweating, dizziness, drowsiness, diarrhea, dry mouth, stomachaches, stomach bloating, etc. Sometimes, soon after a patient with stomachaches takes *da chai hu yang* or *danggui shaoyao san* (whose main ingredients are Angelica sinensis and Chinese herbaceous peony), the stomach can hurt more. Other patients will cough harder after taking medicine, but will feel better afterward.

Antibiotics are mostly cold in nature, according to TCM. When they enter a patient's body along with much fluid (water also is cold in nature), it can make the patient colder. People who have had infusions know this from their personal experience. If you have fever, coughing, or inflammation of the tonsils, you will feel much better after an infusion. But after a few days' treatment, your body can become weak and cold. Genuine TCM doctors treat such diseases by resuming the *yang* energy in the patient's body. This is the only way to change the nature of the cold-induced diseases.

I believe that the real hope for Chinese Medicine does not depend on more and more drugs or prescriptions. These have never been lacking in the history of Chinese Medicine. Nor does it rely on more TCM doctors and clinics. In a sense, the real sign of hope for Chinese Medicine is that greater numbers of patients are experiencing healing crises after taking Chinese Medicine; and more TCM doctors have patients who feel healing reactions."

This article helps to explain why *PaidaLajin* is so effective. Why did the late TCM master Li Ke support the promotion of *PaidaLajin*? Mostly because of the healing crises and self-healing effects. When Dr. Li Ke himself used medicine to treat patients, they would soon experience healing crises.

During one of my seminars in Switzerland, I met with a number of Swiss TCM doctors who use medicinal herbs to boost *yang* energy in patients. They loved *PaidaLajin*. And I told them, "Both *Paida* and *Lajin* help boost *yang* energy. The only difference is we are not using ginger, cassia twig, or monkshood (medicinal herbs that are hot in nature), but the 'medicine' produced in the human body."

Biochemical Changes During *PaidaLajin*

PaidaLajin directly induces biochemical changes in the body and stimulates endocrine secretions the body needs, including insulin.

Bones play an important role in supporting the body, allowing movement, producing blood cells, storing minerals, and regulating pH values. The latest research shows the skeleton and skeletal muscles also have endocrine functions. An increase in osteocalcin contributes to an increase of insulin and a decrease of blood glucose level; increase of adiponectin prevents the accumulation of fat. Insulin is a hormone that lowers blood sugar in the body. It is a major contributor to synthesis of substances in vivo, hence the name 'storage hormone'. Insulin not only regulates sugar metabolism, it also plays an irreplaceable role in the metabolism of fat, water, protein, and trace elements.

Professor Gerard Karsenty of Columbia University and his co-researchers found that osteoblasts (single nucleus cells that synthesize bone) exert an endocrine regulation of the physiological state of other tissues, and that osteocalcin might be one of the hormones directly involved in the process.

The findings had an important clinical implication. It established an entirely new theory for the clinical treatment of diabetes, supported by experimental results. The findings foretold a new therapy for diabetes would be found in the foreseeable future. There could be no better news for diabetic patients. Diabetics and scientists across the world were taking note and anticipating the results eagerly, confident a fresh therapy for diabetes would soon emerge.

Soon after, I began to promote self-healing with *PaidaLajin*. The hundreds of workshops we have held worldwide, and thousands of testimonials of patients' self-healing diabetes with *PaidaLajin*, provide substantial clinical evidence of this new theory. *PaidaLajin* also has a sound scientific interpretation.

Of the various muscles, skeletal muscles (also called striated muscles) are very special. There are over 600 skeletal muscles in the human body, most of which are attached to bones. Bodily movements are performed by contracting and relaxing these muscles.

Skeletal muscles have long been regarded as effector muscles, regulated by the nervous system and bodily fluids. In recent years, a number of experiments have shown skeletal muscles—which make up 40% of your body weight—could be an important, or even the largest, endocrine organ. It secretes, expresses, and synthesizes a variety of biological signaling molecules, including regulatory peptides, cytokines, and growth factors.

1. *Paida* on the joints and bony regions of the body stimulates skeletal muscles.
2. Stretching on a *Lajin* bench stretches all skeletal muscles, and the stimulation can be more intense than yoga and running.
3. *Lajin* sessions can last up to forty minutes per leg.
4. Although the body remains static, *Lajin* strongly stimulates *qi* and blood flow.

5. *PaidaLajin* strongly stimulates the perichondrium and skeletal muscles. During this process, pain and other sensations are felt.
6. The body produces various endocrine secretions specific to individual needs, including stem cells, insulin, adrenaline, enkephalin, and other hormones.

As *PaidaLajin* stimulates specific endocrine secretions, activates the self-healing power, and enhances immunity, it is only natural it can heal chronic diseases. By practicing *PaidaLajin*, a diabetic patient can produce insulin; a menopausal woman can produce needed hormones; and patients with other diseases can produce stem cells, adrenaline, endorphin, and enkephalin. The physical, chemical, and biological transformation process varies from person to person. Chinese Medicine states the body produces endogenous medicine. It is precisely geared to the specific problem and is created with proper stimulation. Such endogenous medicine has no toxic side effects. We can call it organic healing.

New scientific evidence and practical *PaidaLajin* unveil the magic of the self-healing power to everyone, providing healing, weight loss, enhanced cognition and fertility. It can help facilitate natural labor and child-rearing.

Electromagnetic Changes During *PaidaLajin*

Doctors of Western Medicine are educated about the chemical body, and drugs are prescribed to rectify its malfunctions. Based on the "Theory of a Complex System," Professor Changlin Zhang used non-destructive wave detection equipment and discovered, "In addition to the chemical body, there exists an electromagnetic body, and in my opinion, it plays a role of equal or possibly greater importance. It represents an unknown territory in our bodies that now lies within the reach of modern science. Having moved from the realms of mystical experience, science fiction, or pure speculation, it is becoming an important area of basic scientific research in biology and medicine.

"The electromagnetic body is much more complicated and dynamic than the chemical one. If we were able to see it, it would appear completely different to the visible chemical body. We would observe the seven major chakras along the central line of the body and many small chakras in other places emanating various colors. We would see dozens of acupuncture meridians, hundreds of acupuncture points, and numerous micro-acupuncture meridians and points weaving into an intricate network—a continuous interference pattern that is holographic in appearance. Around the body we would discern the aura, as described in ancient beliefs. It exists to some extent in the detectable range of extra-weak light, as well as in the infrared and microwave parts of the electro-magnetic spectrum. Modern technology has seen this become a new area of serious scientific research.

"In addition to being highly complex, the electromagnetic body is also extremely dynamic. Unlike the chemical body, where the bones, organs, vessels, and fibers have fixed positions, definite volumes, and distinct boundaries, the electromagnetic 'organs', such as chakras, and some invisible 'vessels', such as acupuncture meridians, exhibit only a relatively stable position with nebulous boundaries and variable volumes. They are continuously flashing and exhibit continuous changes in intensity, color, and shape, like the surface of the ocean in a fierce storm. This turbulence is particularly evident when the person is experiencing an intense change of emotions and psychological states.

"If we were able to perceive the electromagnetic field in greater detail, we would witness tremendously complicated communication processes being performed at extremely fast speeds. Electromagnetic waves and photons facilitate communication inside the cells, between cells, between bodies, and with the surroundings. All this occurs in addition to the communication occurring through nerve fibers, hormones, and other molecules. As with wireless communication and television broadcasting, communication through electromagnetic fields carries much more information over much wider channels than can be transmitted through insulated nerve fibers and the slow interaction between the surfaces of molecules. Thus, communication within the electromagnetic body has a more profound and subtle influence on our bodies and health."

According to Professor Zhang's research, the dissipative structure of the electromagnetic body is unstable. It is constantly vibrating and has no clear boundaries. Its anatomical features are invisible to the naked eye. The physiological feature of the human body is holographic and indivisible.

The vital feature is that the electromagnetic body governs the chemical body. Reorganizing the former leads to reconstructing the latter. As it relates to pathology, the electromagnetic body is directly influenced by changes in its boundaries.

PaidaLajin is the simplest way of changing the boundaries, leading to the subsequent transformation of the chemical body. The order of the life structure is reorganized, balancing matter and energy, rules and freedom.

PaidaLajin Induces Vibration Changes

The pain caused by *PaidaLajin* stimulates the heart to change its frequency, leading to changes in the frequencies of all organs and cells.

This is consistent with the above-explained Theory of Vibration.

There is limited physical damage to the parts stimulated by *PaidaLajin*.

Normally, a lot of negative charge exists in lumps, toxins, tumors, and inflamed tissue. *PaidaLajin* produces positive charge, which neutralizes the negative charge, decomposing toxins, tumors, and other pathogenic substances. It contributes to *yin-yang* balance.

The process of *PaidaLajin* produces a dialogue between the body and the mind.

PaidaLajin produces the right resonance between them and is conducive to self-healing. Oneness is perfect harmony of the body, mind, and soul.

Energy Boosts During *PaidaLajin*

PaidaLajin boosts energy, both at the stimulated areas and over the entire body, addressing both illness and aging.

In general, the more painful *PaidaLajin* is, the faster internal heat is being produced. We often see people stretched on *Lajin* benches sweating heavily, although they are lying motionless, sometimes even in cold weather.

Where does the boosted energy come from? From the wastes, toxins, and other pathogenic substances are burned, leading to detoxification, enhanced *qi* and blood flow, healing, and weight reduction.

Clinical Explanations

PaidaLajin creates *sha*, swelling, and elongated tendons.

Chinese Medicine believes the human body is like a pharmaceutical factory—it produces whatever medicine it needs. Many people know this theory but are unaware of the details.

Normally, there is pain and swelling during *PaidaLajin*. Persistent pain and swelling indicates continuous detoxification. How fast the pain and swelling fades depends on how smoothly energy flows in the meridian system. When *PaidaLajin* stimulates a specific region of the body, the Heart instantly feels the stimulation. The power is awakened and enhanced rapidly, and it goes on to effect other organs, leading to structural and biochemical changes in the entire body. This war heals various disorders—physical, mental, and psychological.

According to Chinese Medicine, there are two major causes of illness:

1. Excessive desires and emotions.
2. Discord between the body's internal and external environments.

PaidaLajin regulates and balances both.

Both the theory of Chinese Medicine and recent advancements in Western medical science help us better identify the root causes of illness. People used to disregard the connection between excessive emotions and diseases until psychosomatic medicine emerged in the past two or three decades. Psychosomatic medicine posits that over a thousand diseases, including tumors, diabetes, and hypertension, are caused by negative emotions accumulated and trapped in the body over time. This produced an interdisciplinary approach to illness. It also provides a good example of scientific development testifying to the wisdom of Chinese Medicine.

PaidaLajin, the self-help slapping and stretching exercises handed down from ancient times, re-emerges before us and fills this gap. We can use the theory of Chinese Medicine to clearly explain how and why it works. But we also need to explain it concisely in scientific language, so people of our contemporary era can better comprehend it.

***Yang* energy:**

- Decomposes fat
- Lowers the blood lipid level
- Enhances the cardiac systolic function
- Accelerates the decomposition of glycogen
- Dilates the blood vessels of the heart, liver, bones, tendons, and ligaments
- Expands the windpipe

- Increases oxygen supply
- Causes your body to secrete more insulin, osteocalcin, and vascular angiotensin
- Helps you to slim down
- Lowers your blood glucose levels
- Enhances metabolism of fat, sugar, water, protein, and trace elements

PaidaLajin Stimulates Stem Cell Production

PaidaLajin not only stimulates your skin, nerves, and subcutaneous blood vessels, it also has a strong impact on your bones, skeletal muscles, tendons, and ligaments.

Normally, you mainly slap joints. This induces production of stem cells in the perichondrium of the joints.

Stem cells:

1. Seem to infinitely proliferate and multi-directionally differentiate. This means they can copy themselves and change their nature.
2. Engage in immune and hematopoietic (blood-building) activities.
3. Are self-replicable.
4. They play a vital role in repairing pathological damages to organs and tissues.

Many medical theories and treatments underline the importance of stem cells. During the body's re-organization process, old and damaged organs and cells are replaced, recovering physiological functions. It can be called an autologous (self-generated) stem cell regeneration.

Jin includes all elastic connective tissues that link the skeleton, muscles, and organs:

- Tendons
- Ligaments
- Fascia
- Cartilage

Lajin not only impacts the connective tissue, it also stimulates the skeleton, fascia, and muscles. There are tendons on bones and muscles, as well as on organs. *Lajin* stimulates them all. The ancient Chinese classics *Yi Jin Jing* (The Classic of Tendon-Muscle Strengthening Exercises) and *Xi Sui Jing* (The Classic of Bone Marrow Cleansing) both elaborated on the effect of stretching.

PaidaLajin Increases Body Temperature

Paida and *Lajin* both directly increase body temperature.

Through observation of nature, or according to Chinese and Western Medicine, we know diseases are mostly cold induced. All sorts of viruses, tumors, and blockages are caused by cold-related stagnation. During the aging process, the body temperature drops continually, as circulation becomes less efficient. When a person dies, the body cools down completely.

PaidaLajin noticeably increases your body temperature, locally and holistically. This is the natural result when the innate self-healing power is strengthened. Your inner vitality is rejuvenated and enhanced. Your body's capacity to produce heat makes you more disease-resistant and gives you anti-aging abilities.

Conclusion

In the healthcare sector, we all strive for positive curative effects. The message of *PaidaLajin* is being shared rapidly in the online world, benefiting more and more people all the time. An increasing number of hospitals, yoga schools, temples, monasteries, and health and meditation centers are teaching *PaidaLajin.*

All of the claims have been measured and evaluated using modern scientific methods and devices, based on medical standards. Whether experts believe and test it or not, the great mass movement of self-healing with *PaidaLajin* is unstoppable. Attracted by the obvious interests in self-healing, more and more people around the world are voluntarily practicing and sharing *PaidaLajin*. Precisely because it is a non-medical therapy, it makes up for what is lacking in the medical world.

In the final analysis, *PaidaLajin* is a way of life.

Extracellular Matrix (ECM) Regulation

Founded by Viennese anatomist Alfred Pischinger and his colleagues, ECM regulation presents a theory that helps us understand *PaidaLajin* more clearly.

Every cell requires a suitable environment called the ground substance, or ECM, for successful microcirculation. ECM is closely connected with the hormonal and nervous systems, including the brain. The communication network of the above-mentioned systems, and all of the connected organs, is known as the system of extracellular matrix regulation.

"Stated simply, every function and every process in the living body involves the matrix in one way or another. Every cell in the body is nourished via the matrix, and all waste products of cellular metabolism pass through the ground substance, which is the actual environment. The matrix is also the terrain in which all immune responses and tissue repair processes take place.

"The matrix is not an inert filler substance or filter but is instead a body-wide communication and support system, vital to all functions.

"Both Western biomedicine and all of the Eastern therapies find a valuable common denominator in the study of the ground matrix

system. For it is in the matrix that the causes and cures of systemic and chronic illness can be found."

These are the words from pages XII and XIII of the book *The Extracellular Matrix and Ground Regulation*. Many therapies have been used to achieve long-lasting changes to ECM regulation, such as acupuncture, massage, magnetic fields, and local anesthetics. Many difficult diseases were healed. This is what they have in common:

1. They all stimulate skin or tissue; connective tissue plays a major role.
2. Any stimulus exceeding a particular low-intensity threshold will trigger a reaction in the entire matrix.
3. They are done by professionals and applied to the connected areas.
4. They are referred to as a complementary medicine, intended to be combined with major therapies.

As for *PaidaLajin*, it also stimulates the skin and other tissue, but the intensity is much stronger. Yet it can be controlled by each individual. *PaidaLajin* can be achieved by anyone after learning the basics by reading the book, attending a workshop, or engaging in an online course. Most importantly, *PaidaLajin* is not a complementary treatment, but a lifestyle change. It's not a therapy or a medicine. The degrees of treatment and the session times are flexible and controllable. At home or at a workshop, you may do it eight to ten hours a day, though this is harder to achieve at home. The treatment is under everyone's control.

How does it work?

(From Page 7 of the ECM book):

"In contrast to the classical closed, Newtonian system, the open system (i.e. matrix) shows that when suitable energy is supplied (non-chaotic energy), it can instantly spread throughout the entire system. In an autocatalytic manner (acting as its own catalyst), this leads to the appearances of new structures, and these can develop further into a higher structural order."

This is why we say *PaidaLajin* is self-healing: it happens automatically.

The meridian theory and points used in acupuncture can be used in *PaidaLajin* as well.

1. Every slap covers more than one meridian or one acupuncture point. It's normal to cover three meridians and more than five points when slapping.
2. Slapping on a local area can last from one minute to an hour.
3. The intensity can be much stronger than one needle, causing more stimulation.
4. Slapping on skin can penetrate so deeply it reaches tissue, muscles, vessels, capillaries, bones, cells, ligaments, nerves, and—of course, ECM—and this strongly and holistically impacts the whole body.
5. Lajin shares the same characteristics with *Paida*, through powerfully stretching ligaments and tissue.
6. Pain plays a big role in communication between the systems and organs via ECM. As pain varies in degree and locations, it can be used in both diagnosing and healing, by controlling *PaidaLajin's* intensity and duration.
7. In contrast to covering up symptoms, *PaidaLajin* uncovers known and unknown diseases, and heals them at the same time it reveals them. This is a very unique phenomenon from *PaidaLajin* and Traditional Chinese Medicine (TCM.)

(From Page 3 from the ECM book):

"Focusing on an illness, according to its type, replaces the individual phenomenon of being sick. Turning this disease into a model makes it accessible to instrumental measurements in a causal-analytical way. Reality is replaced by models, and the more complex the reality is, the more simplified the models become. A model offers neither the framework for determining individual biological outcomes or their quality of life."

Please note that *PaidaLajin* focuses on tissue, which is the key to understanding why one simple method can heal so many different diseases. Like the meridian theory presented in TCM, the ECM presents an answer for healing by traditional Western Medicine.

(From Page 3 of the ECM book):

"It has been known for a long time that the tissue in question forms the basis of the entire body. Figuratively, it is also the ground in which all organs take root. To a certain extent, it is both ground and matrix. It has its own essential value ... the functional connections between the capillary bed and the cells are through the extracellular matrix, whose disruption is the starting point of diseases ... the many processes and presentations that are involved in healthy and pathological events of the physical body are nothing more than variations of one and the same basic physiological process—variations in metabolism and in every exchange; variations of stage and site (the Law of Stages.) With this, Ricker was able to confirm the experiential medicine passed on by Hippocrates, Galen, Paracelsus, and Hahnemann. According to all of them, diseases are similar, and the dose is the healing factor, not the specific substance. As it has been demonstrated by experience, a curative dose of one remedy has the ability to cure many diseases."

Because the healing of *PaidaLajin* is instantaneous, it quickly spread throughout the world. In some places, entire families—or even whole communities or villages—do it. As it continues to spread, more data will be on record. There is a strange phenomenon: professional medical institutions don't conduct any clinical research on *PaidaLajin*, and thus have no recorded accounts, yet thousands of reports appear every day from normal people around the world.

For more information about ECM and holistic healing, I suggest you read *The Extracellular Matrix and Ground Regulation*. The author is Alfred Pischinger, and it was published by North Atlantic Books.

I owe a debt of gratitude to Dr. Pischinger and to Dr. Hartmut Heine, who edited the book, and Ingeborg Eibl, who translated it from German into English. I feel like we are a team. We, the everyday people, have done the clinical trials on hundreds of diseases, and Dr. Pischinger and his colleagues have done the theory and lab research. They have tried multiple means of stimulating ECM, but they haven't tested *PaidaLajin* yet. Once they do, I am sure they will have more amazing discoveries to share.

Effectiveness Rates of *PaidaLajin* on Patients with Diabetes and Hypertension (2010)

The second workshop in Beijing was held November 17–23, 2010.

Six participants were diabetic, and thirteen had abnormal blood pressure levels.

All voluntarily stopped medication and insulin, and *PaidaLajin* was 100% effective in improving their conditions. One participant who suffered from low blood pressure found it rose up to a healthy level.

Statistics for Diabetic Patients

During the workshop, participants jogged in the morning, did *PaidaLajin* for four to five hours a day, fasted for three days, and drank ginger and jujube tea with brown sugar in it.

Blood Glucose Levels Before & After *PaidaLajin*

Name Gender Age	**Symptoms and Medication Before Workshop**	**Average Level Daily**	**Level Before *PaidaLajin***	**Level After *PaidaLajin***
Zhu Female 65	Diabetic for six years, had hypoglycemic drugs and insulin injections: Acarbose, one tablet/time, three times a day; Hydrochloride Enteric-coated Tablets, two tablets/time, three times a day; Betahistine, two tablets /day; Insulin injection 9 units/time, once a day	9.4	November 16 16 17:00: 9.4	Stopped medication on November 17 November 22, morning (fasting): 6.3
Lee Male 58	Diabetic for eleven years, had hypoglycemic drugs and supplements: Recovery capsules, Cordyceps capsules, Ginkgo capsules, Alpha capsules, Rhizoma Coptidis capsules, Metformin	8.5-9	November 17, morning (fasting): 6.2	Stopped medication on November 17 November 22, morning (fasting): 5.6
Fan Female 45	Suspected herself of having diabetes, never received treatment or taken medicine for it		November 16, morning (three hours after meal): 8.9	November 22, morning (fasting): 5.3

Blood Glucose Levels Before & After *PaidaLajin*

Name Gender Age	Symptoms and Medication Before Workshop	Average Level Daily	Level Before *PaidaLajin*	Level After *PaidaLajin*
Xiao Male 78	Diabetic for twelve years, had hypoglycemic drugs: Acarbose Tablets, two tablets/time, three times a day	6.5	November 17, morning (fasting): 3.6	Stopped medication on November 17 November 22, morning (fasting): 5.9
Jiang Female 74	No hypoglycemic drugs, had Propolis: two tablets/time, two times/day for a year		November 16, afternoon: 8.3	Stopped medication on November 16 November 22, morning (fasting): 4.8
Liu Female 72	Diabetic for ten years, had hypoglycemic drugs: Dipotassium Hydrochloride Sustained Release Tablets, one tablet/day Acarbose Tablets, 2 tablets/day	Fasting: 7 After meal: 9	November 16, afternoon: 7.2	Stopped medication on November 17 November 22, morning (fasting): 5.5

Statistics for Hypertensive Patients

Blood Pressure Levels Before & After *PaidaLajin*

Name Gender Age	Symptoms and Medication Before Workshop	Blood Pressure mmHg	Symptoms and Medication After Workshop	Blood Pressure mmHg
Zhu, Female, 65	Dizzy	140/70	Dizziness gone	125/80
Dang, Female, 54	None	140/80	None	130/79
Lee, Male, 58	None Taking supplements	90/60	Blood pressure rose to normal Stopped medication on November 17	110/80
Xiao, Female, 67	Swelling discomfort in the head for over ten years, never took medicine for it	160/100	Symptom gone	120/80
Liu, Female, 61	None Never taken medicine for it	140/90	None	125/80
Lee, Male, 65	None	140/98	None	130/80
Zhu, Male, 61	Swelling discomfort in the head, could not sleep well, irregular heartbeat, Nifedipine, two tablets/day 25mmg Aspirin, one tablet/day	170/90	Symptoms improved Stopped medication on November 17	154/100

Statistics for Hypertensive Patients

Blood Pressure Levels Before & After *PaidaLajin*

Name Gender Age	Symptoms and Medication Before Workshop	Blood Pressure mmHg	Symptoms and Medication After Workshop	Blood Pressure mmHg
Xiao, Female, 73	Dizzy, head shaking involuntarily	140/80	Symptoms gone	110/74
Xiao, Male, 78	Dizzy Micardis, one tablet/day	170/80	Symptom gone	120/70
Liu, Female, 72	Dizzy, pain on the right side of the head Nifedipine Controlled Release Tablets, two tablets/day	180/60	Symptoms gone Stopped medication on November 17	150/80
Cao, Male, 74	None No medication	149/90	None	132/80
Lu, Male, 72	Dizzy Nitrendipine, one tablet/day	150/118	Symptom gone Stopped medication on November 17	130/90
Jiang, Female, 74	Swelling discomfort in the head, blurred vision, shed tears involuntarily, hypertensive for ten years Felodipine Sustained Release Tablets, Nitrendipine, one tablet per day for over twenty years	140/80	Symptom gone Stopped medication on November 17	138/80

POST-WORKSHOP SURVEYS

In August 2011, we conducted post-workshop surveys over the phone.

Total Interviews

Of 418 participants, including those who attended more than one workshop, 285 agreed to participate. (68% of participants.) 97 (34%) were male and 188 (66%) were female.

1. Some overseas participants couldn't be reached by phone.
2. Contact information was incorrect or outdated.
3. Several calls weren't answered.

SUMMARY

243 (85%) of them continued *PaidaLajin*. 15% didn't, due to these reasons:

- Too busy
- Felt healthy
- Laziness
- Intolerance of pain
- Switched to other treatments
- Objection from family members
- Insignificant effects

Medication Taken by People Who Continued *PaidaLajin*

226 (93%) stopped medication altogether, while 17 (7%) continued to take medicine. The reasons cited:

"I'm worried I can't be healed with just *PaidaLajin*."

"My doctor asked me to continue medication."

"*PaidaLajin*, combined with medication, can help me more."

Participant Who Stopped Medication and Continued *PaidaLajin*

134 (59%) reported excellent health; 76 participants (34%) saw visible improvements, and the remaining 16 (7%) reported the same health they experienced when previously medicated.

Those who enjoyed excellent health continued *PaidaLajin* and included jogging almost every day.

Further Analysis

a. Sciatica

Ninety-three survey participants suffered from sciatica. Ninety-one of them (98%) reported significant self-healing effects.

b. Diabetes

Twelve out of fourteen survey participants with diabetes reported significant healing.

c. Hypertension

Thirty of the thirty-four survey participants with hypertension reported significant self-healing effects. The four with inconclusive results only did *PaidaLajin* occasionally, and they didn't always take their medication.

PAIDALAJIN CLINICAL RESEARCH WORKSHOP REPORT (2015) TAG-VHS DIABETES RESEARCH CENTRE IN CHENNAI, INDIA

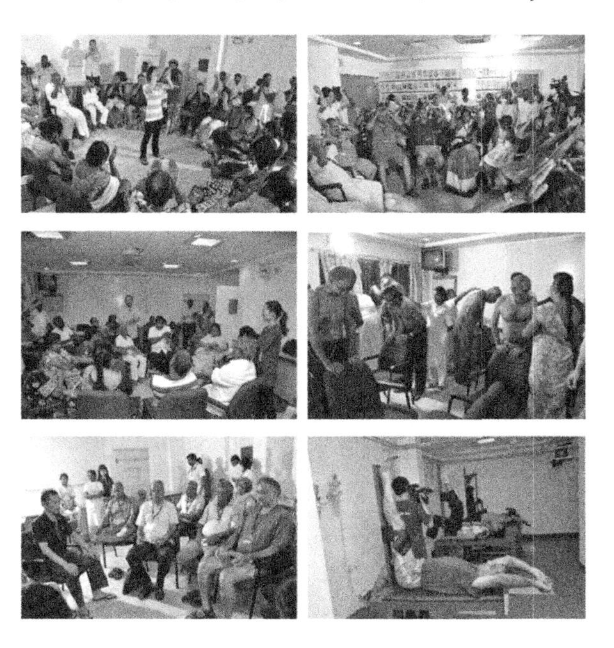

The following is an excerpt from the report. Download the full report on Classroom—Downloads on our English website (http://*paidalajin*.com/en/home.)

SUMMARY

1. A unique clinical research workshop on the Chinese self-healing method termed *PaidaLajin*, promoted by Master Hongchi Xiao, was conducted under continuous strict medical supervision and detailed computerized/video-graphed data recording at the TAG VHS Diabetics Research Centre in Chennai, India from March 9-13, 2015.

2. A total of twenty-five participants were registered for the five-day program, a bridge from the full course of seven days advocated by Master Hongchi Xiao (due to logistic reasons.) He conducted this personally along with his assistants and Indian colleague, Mr. Parag Samel. The entire program started at seven a.m. daily and lasted for almost ten to eleven hours daily with a short break for breakfast & lunch. The entire program was given free of cost to all the participants. About ten of them were in-patients, while the rest came as outpatients. All of them were fully screened medically; their cases documented and after detailed counseling sessions, their informed consent for the entire procedure, including photography, was obtained from all the participants. Five out of the twenty-five registered participants dropped out from the workshop due to compelling personal reasons; we have the entire data of progress for the twenty persons who completed the program successfully.

CONCLUSION

While this abridged *PaidaLajin* workshop done under near-perfect conditions revealed that, though it is not a Panacea for all illnesses, it could nevertheless prove to be a veritable blessing to prevent illness and promote good health, enthusiasm, and energy to every individual practicing this self-healing method diligently, with faith and trust in the WISDOM OF THE HUMAN BODY GIFTED TO HUMANKIND BY THE UNIVERSAL LIFE FORCE. (GOD!)

The following are several take-home messages from the workshop:

1. Type II Diabetes responds very well to *PaidaLajin* therapy in the holistic workshop setting. This is not surprising as it involves a very strict diet regime, fasting, and control of mind and through shot/effective sessions of medications. A dedicated and motivated ex-soldier normalized his established diabetes without any of the medications he had taken previously during this short span of five days and remains in excellent health more than a week after leaving the workshop. This definitely raises hope for newly/recently (< one year) detected Type II Diabetes to try out this regime for at least three to six months. There is promise that all cases of IGT and many cases of overt asymptomatic Type II Diabetes could use this modality as the first choice for benefits.

2. Type I Diabetes (Juvenile Insulin-Dependent Diabetes Mellitus) which is the more severe, insulinopenic form, occurring in children and young adolescents, also recorded improvement during the clinical condition over the five-day period of the workshop; however, during the healing crisis (healing reactions) and fasting when their blood sugars went up, they needed medical support in the form of calories, fluid, and small doses of rapid-acting insulin to prevent ketoacidosis. It was not alarming and all of them recovered and completed the full course with renewed energy, needing approximately half of their original requirement of insulin. A longer period of observation (six months) is underway, which may provide more answers.

3. Hypertension was not an issue at all during the entire duration for any of those patients who were on varying doses of anti-hypertensive medication. After one week of returning home, only one out of ten

people who were taking medication required half of the original dose. Even this needs review and revision with continuation of therapy.

4. There were four persons with varying labels of coronary artery disease/ischemic heart disease. None of them had any problems during the strenuous workshop. It is too short a period to assess the impact of *PaidaLajin* on heart disease. We need to study a much larger sample, over a longer time period, to assess the full benefits claimed for this condition.

5. A host of minor and chronic illnesses like knee pains (OA), hip pains (OA), low backache, periarthritis of shoulders, degenerative painful diseases of the spine (spondylitis), and disc bulges were treated with ease and assurance with a remarkably high percentage of success (98%.)

6. The true discovery and revaluation of *PaidaLajin* during this study was its remarkable, almost dramatic improvement, in cases of Parkinsonism, facilitating reduction in one and complete withdrawal of anti-Parkinson's drug in the other case. This provides a definite silver lining to the millions of patients around the world afflicted with many types of Parkinsonism and the resultant drug-induced dyskinesias and other ADR. The mobility offered after *PaidaLajin* was unparalleled and exciting to watch/demonstrate (video graphs.) Surely this workshop has shown that there is hope and optimism for patients with Parkinson's disease. A systematic, large, and long-term study for about three years will, I believe, reveal all the benefits that might qualitatively improve their lives.

7. The final take-home message of *PaidaLajin* workshop was, indeed, that it virtually doubled the ENERGY LEVELS of all the participants (100%), both individually and as a mass effect. It gave optimism and hope to all the persons involved with the idea of health taking precedence over disease, self-healing taking lead over seeking

medication, and fear of the unknown/imaginary risks giving way to self-confidence in these simple methods of self-healing.

CLINICAL REPORT: TWO PARKINSON'S PATIENTS DURING AND AFTER A WORKSHOP IN INDIA (2015) BY THE TAG-VHS DIABETES RESEARCH CENTRE IN CHENNAI, INDIA

Parkinsonism

ID: 3975 – (Marks: 5/10)

This fifty-eight-year old man with H/o. Parkinsonism under treatment came to our center recently for initiation of Pulsed Electromagnetic Field Energy Therapy, using a BM Pulser. He is a known case of T2DM – eight years / HTN – five years on medical management. His main complaints are rigidity left upper limb ++, eye movement upward gaze present, downward gaze absent, and tends to lean on the left side. He also had aphonia (a barely audible voice.) He is on Tab. Syndopa plus 100/25 four times a day. He completed the five-day course. His rigidity reduced significantly, and his blood sugar was well under control without OHA. He could phonate audibly. His anti-Parkinsonism drug dosage was reduced by 50% and anti-BP medicines were stopped for the time being.

He is following the *PaidaLajin* self-healing therapy at home and feels improvement with rigidity. Sugars were also well controlled without OHA.

ID: 1653 – (Marks: 9/10)

This seventy-three-year-old man is our TAG VHS DRC-registered patient for the last two and a half years. He is a known case of Parkinsonism—seven years, on medical management (Tab. Syndopa plus 125 mg five times a day) + Pulsed Electromagnetic Field Energy Therapy, using a BM Pulser. He showed only slight improvement. Sometimes he was not able to walk, had slurred speech on and off, and was not able to turn quickly. He participated in the five-day clinical workshop. Every day, he showed significant improvement. After five days, his speech was clear, he was able to walk without support, his limbs were supple, and he exhibited all-round improvements in his physical condition. This case was truly remarkable, as the *PaidaLajin* therapy facilitated drug withdrawal completely. To the best of our knowledge, in medical literature, no other non-drug therapy has been known to facilitate complete drug withdrawal for an established case of Parkinsonism of a long duration!

He is following *PaidaLajin* self-healing therapy at home and feels remarkable improvement in gait and walk.

The following are The Hindu report and pictures of improvement in a Parkinson's patient before and after *Paida*:

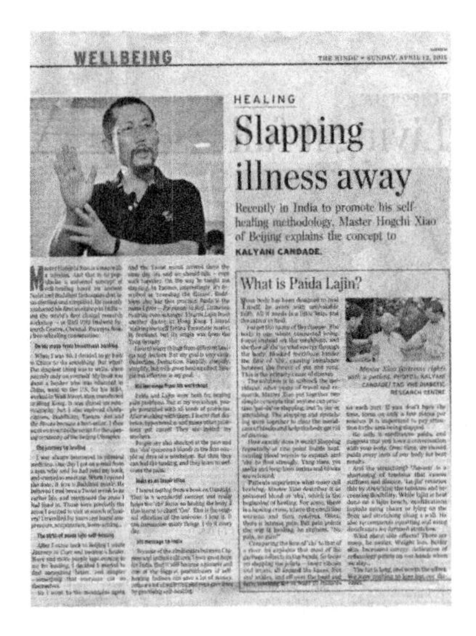

WELLBEING

HEALING

Slapping illness away

Recently in India to promote his self-healing methodology, Master Hogchi Xiao of Beijing explains the concept to KALYANI CANDADE.

What is Paida Lajin?

THE HINDU
(paper version)
Slapping Illness Away

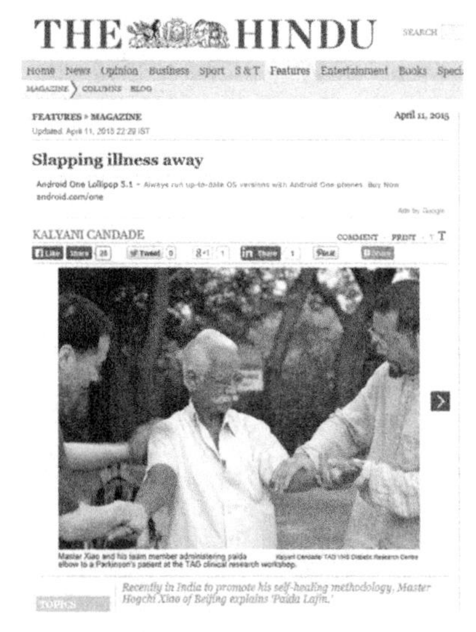

THE HINDU

Home News Opinion Business Sport S&T Features Entertainment Books

MAGAZINE COLUMNS BLOG

FEATURES › MAGAZINE

April 11, 2015

Slapping illness away

KALYANI CANDADE

Master Xiao and his team member administering paida elbow to a Parkinson's patient at the TAG clinical research workshop.

Recently in India to promote his self-healing methodology, Master Hogchi Xiao of Beijing explains 'Paida Lajin.'

THE HINDU
(online version)
Slapping Illness Away

Administering *Paida* to the Elbows of a Parkinson's patient atthe TAG Clinical Research Workshop.

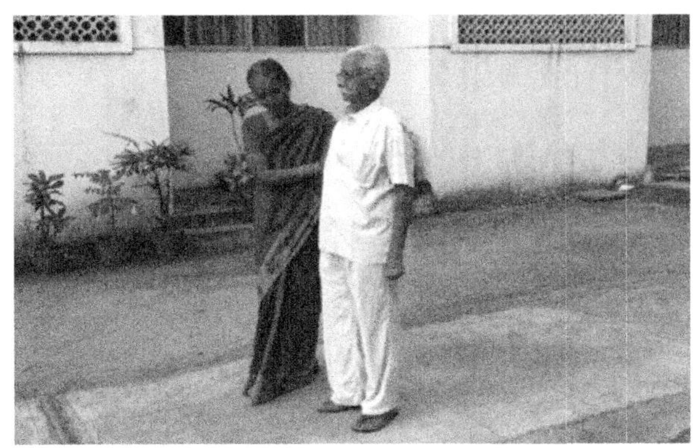

Before *Paida*, the patient could only take very small steps due to stiff legs.

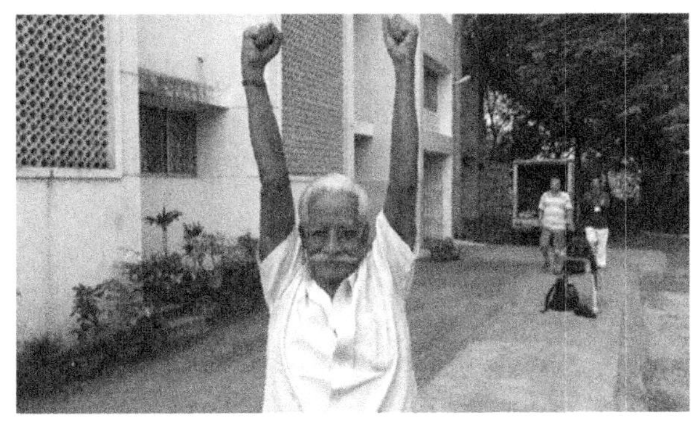

Improved arm and leg mobility after *Paida*.

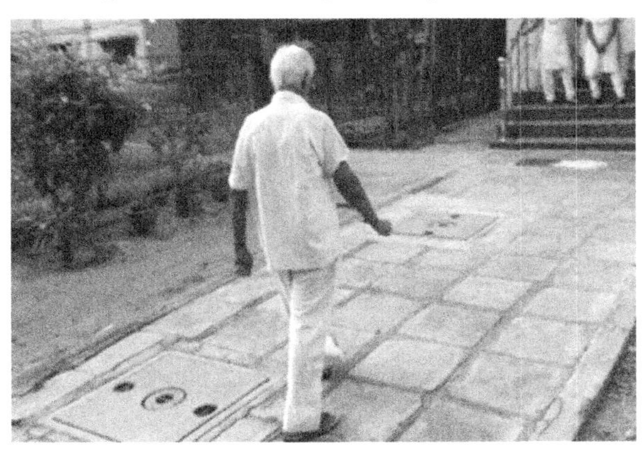

After being slapped on his inner elbows, he was able to make big strides and walk up the stairs without support.

As the Internet and wearable devices become more popular around the world, it will be easier to measure personal health data. In the future, big data sets from more *PaidaLajin* users will attest to the healing effects. It will be a new era. I call it The Era of Self-Healing.

HEALING EFFECTS

Dealing with *Sha*

Continue *Paida* until *sha* fades away. This is called Thorough *Paida*.

The color will deepen as you continue, but eventually it will get lighter and fade away. Soon your skin will look normal again. You can see for yourself by comparing *sha* on your arms or knees. Continue *Paida* on only one side. The *sha* receiving continuous *Paida* will heal faster.

Some people use moxibustion, acupuncture, bloodletting, or cupping to speed up the process of healing. We recommend continued *PaidaLajin*. It is the simplest, most convenient, and most effective method.

Bathing in a hot spring will soothe the pain and heal *sha* faster.

ADVICE ABOUT SHARING *PAIDALAJIN*

Advice for *PaidaLajin* Promoters:

1. You might be excited to share, but it's a good idea to wait until you know more.
2. Many people haven't practiced enough, and they lack the experience to answer questions and address the different possible reactions.
3. Only tell people who are interested in learning more. Don't force it on anyone or encourage them to stop medication or other medical services.

4. Practice a lot before you tell anyone else. Carefully read *PaidaLajin* Self-Healing, most of the articles on our website, and attend a seven-day workshop. You need to understand the physical and psychological changes people will go through before you advise them. They might ask challenging questions you can't answer.

5. Don't practice *PaidaLajin* too intensely. It's easy to try to rush the process, and it can turn others away from the practice before they begin.

6. Clearly explain the concept and phenomena of healing reactions and how to deal with them. Explain they are inevitable during diagnosis and detoxification, and they are positive signs. They will otherwise see rewards as punishments. If they speak to doctors who don't understand *PaidaLajin*, it can lead to even more confusion.

7. *Sha* isn't the only way to judge the effectiveness of *Paida*.

8. Ensure they know to continue *Paida* until *sha* disappears.

9. Everyone's pain tolerance is different. Don't make assumptions about other people. Reduce the intensity if they request it.

10. If someone asks you a question you can't answer, don't try. Advise them to read the book and visit our websites.

11. Practicing and understanding *PaidaLajin* isn't enough. You need to back up your practice with a good diet and other good health habits.

12. Nourish your own Heart before advising other people. Self-healing is the holistic healing of your body, mind, and soul. You need to heal yourself first.

REMINDERS

1. *Paida* and *Lajin* are self-healing methods. You can use *PaidaLajin* on yourself or others. When helping others, please ask for their permission BEFORE you do it.
2. Generally speaking, go gradually from soft to heavy. In emergencies, use heavy slaps right away.
3. Hot, cold, sore, numb, itchy, painful, tingling, and/or swelling can happen during and after *PaidaLajin*. Patches of red, purple, blue, and/or black can appear at the slapped areas. Rashes, burping, flatulence, and dark and stinky urine and feces may result. These are good reactions. There is no need to worry.
4. Stay warm and avoid cold and wind during and after *PaidaLajin*.
5. Both laypersons and doctors have personally experienced instant, miraculous effects in relieving acute symptoms. In case of an emergency, don't panic or wait for help. All you need is a pair of hands and a caring heart—dedicated to saving yourself or someone else.
6. According to legal provisions in many countries, in an emergency, first aid can be provided without a doctor's license.
7. This is for your reference only. The decision to practice *PaidaLajin* is at your discretion, and you are responsible for any and all consequences.

18

OTHER *QI* EXERCISES AND MEDITATION

WAIST SWIRLING

Waist swirling is easy to learn and produces quick results. You can practice it anytime and anywhere. It boosts kidney energy, and helps relieve urinary, digestive, reproductive, and gynecological disorders. It also helps you lose weight around your belly, waist, and buttocks.

1. Stand with your feet shoulders-width apart. Cling your toes tightly to the ground. Slightly bend your torso forward.
2. Bend your elbows at about ninety degrees. Place your hands below your belly button, with your palms facing inward. Stretch open your fingers as much as possible, and use your thumbs and index fingers to form an empty diamond. (This keeps your shoulders in place during the exercise.)
3. With your spine at the center, make your buttocks and waist swirl to the left, back, right, and front sides. Do a 360-degree circle. While swirling your waist, keep your shoulders, elbows, and hands in the same place. Swirl twenty times, then swirl twenty times in the other direction. Repeat this for five to fifteen minutes a day.
4. Open your mouth slightly. Inhale through your nose and exhale through your mouth and nose at the same time.

After a few minutes, you will feel achy, and your spine will get warmer and warmer.

Notes:

- Make sure you stretch your fingers as much as possible.
- Swirl only your waist and hips, keeping everything else in place.
- Keep your toes clinging to the ground the whole time. This will fix your position, absorb energy from the Earth, and clear meridian blockages in your feet.

TIE QIANG GONG

This is a secret therapy that boosts kidney energy. Within a few minutes, your waist, kidneys, and entire spine will warm up.

1. Stand facing a wall.
2. Set your feet shoulders-width apart.
3. Touch the tip of your nose and toes to the wall.
4. Slowly squat down, keeping your nose on the wall.
5. Go all the way down, until your legs are bent and folded together.
6. Hug your legs with your arms.
7. Keep your nose against the wall.
8. Slowly stand up, keeping your nose against the wall.
9. Repeat the same exercise.

A man over seventy suffered from fatigue, tinnitus, prostatitis, kidney deficiency, and persistent insomnia. He tried many treatments, but all to no avail. After practicing *tie qiang gong* for less than two months, his hearing and prostate problems were gone, and he slept much better.

It is even better to combine *tie qiang gong*, *PaidaLajin*, and waist swirling.

Notes:

Begin cautiously. You can move your feet away from the wall for balance. Make sure your spine is straight and your body is stable.

It's recommended you do it in multiples of nine (nine, eighteen, twenty-four, thirty-six, etc.) There is no limit.

WALL HITTING

Wall hitting is a secret therapy derived from *t'ai chi*. For many people, *t'ai chi* can be too difficult to learn. Wall hitting is a simple practice.

Caution: Do not practice if you are pregnant, or have injuries or unhealed wounds on your back.

Philosophy and Effect

Similar to *PaidaLajin*, wall hitting can heal many things, but it isn't a guaranteed cure for everything.

From the perspective of Chinese Medicine, wall hitting stimulates the Du Meridian along the spine and the Urinary Bladder Meridian on either side of it. The energy travels up the Du Meridian to the head. When the body leaves the wall, the energy goes down the Ren Meridian along the front middle of the torso. The energy flow completes a full cycle in the body.

Because the urinary bladder is paired with the kidneys, stimulating the Urinary Bladder Meridian helps enhance kidney function. Also, acupoints along the Urinary Bladder Meridian are linked to other internal organs.

From the perspectives of *qi gong*, *t'ai chi*, and Chinese Medicine, wall hitting creates an energy field around the entire body. The energy is both inside and outside, regulating *yin-yang* and the internal organs. A *t'ai chi* practitioner aims not for greater physical strength, but for a higher energy level. Similarly, we practice wall hitting to boost energy. A *t'ai chi* master once said, "Wall hitting creates a protective shield around us. It is particularly useful for improving stomach and intestine functions, and facilitating bowel movements."

From the perspective of Western Medicine, wall hitting stimulates all the internal organs, and the body will produce many stem cells and endocrine secretions such as insulin, endorphins, and dopamine that the body needs for self-healing. It also creates a healing vibration that impacts all the organs and cells, thus helping to clear acids and wastes in the body. It facilitates cell activation and regeneration, enhances immune, urinary and reproductive functions, and heals diseases—either directly or indirectly.

From the perspective of anatomy, the entire spine vibrates during wall hitting. It adjusts dislocated joints, tendons, ligaments, and other soft tissues connected to the spine. It relieves pressure on the nerves. Like *Lajin*, it helps with bones setting.

Because the spinal cord is linked to the brain, wall hitting stimulates all the nerves, meridians, and blood vessels associated with the brain. This is helpful for cerebrovascular diseases.

Wall hitting relaxes back muscles, improving circulation and metabolism.

1. Stand with your back facing a solid wall.
2. Set your feet shoulder-width apart. The distance between your feet and the wall should be about 1.5 times the length of your shoe.
3. Tighten your leg muscles to stay steady.
4. Slightly drop your buttocks.
5. Cross your arms around your chest, or let your arms hang down naturally.
6. Inhale deeply through your nose.
7. Let your body fall back onto the wall. The moment your back hits the wall, your back and internal organs are massaged. Exhale through your nose and mouth.

8. Don't hold your breath. You can open your mouth all of the way if necessary.
9. Stick out your buttocks so your shoulder blades don't hit the wall first. Your entire back should hit the wall at the same time.
10. Keep both feet on the ground.
11. If you know which meridian is blocked or where you feel pain, focus on hitting that part against the wall.
12. Stand further away from the wall to increase the intensity of the exercise.

Note:

Use a strong, load-bearing wall with a flat, smooth surface. Otherwise you could injure yourself.

You can practice wall hitting one to three times a day, hitting the wall 200–1,000 times during each session. This should take ten minutes to two hours.

Similar to *PaidaLajin*, you might burp and or pass gas. You may experience headaches, dizziness, neck pain, stomachache, or pain in your tailbone. These indicate lurking problems in your body.

You can watch videos of wall hitting, waist swirling, and *tie qiang gong* exercises in the video section of our website: http://www.*paidala-jin*.com/en/home.

ZEN JOGGING

Zen jogging is a form of meditation.

1. Make fists. Hide your thumbs inside your other fingers.
2. Empty your mind and lower your head. Look at your feet the whole time and begin to slowly jog.
3. Follow the rhythm with your breathing.

4. If you are gasping, slow down. It's OK to move even slower than walking. The key is to stay focused on jogging and breathing. Please do not walk. You'll lose the vibrations, and your feet won't receive *Paida*.
5. Zen jog for thirty to sixty minutes. You'll sweat a bit, but you'll feel refreshed instead of tired.
6. In the warm days of spring, summer, and fall, practice barefoot jogging. It helps you absorb the energy from the Earth.
7. Zen jogging may feel unpleasant first, but you'll adjust with practice.

BREATHING EXERCISES

1. Inhale slowly and fully into your abdomen through your nose.
2. Hold your breath for three to fifty seconds, and exhale quickly through your mouth.
3. Do this 50–500 times a day. As you practice, you will be able to hold your breath for longer than fifty seconds.
4. Practice this while doing *PaidaLajin*, and during other times in the day.
5. This can rapidly improve spleen and kidney energy.
6. Insomnia, dizziness, a runny nose, and pins and needles are natural. You can help relieve them by slapping your inner elbows.

MEDITATION

Meditation nourishes the Heart. It heals physical, mental, and psychological problems—and leads the way to enlightenment. It is more difficult than *PaidaLajin*. In our workshops, we meditate twice a day.

People tend to associate meditation with religion, but it no longer has religious barriers. It is now widely accepted and practiced around the world. There are also scientific studies that show the practical benefits of meditation.

If you have your own method of meditation, continue to practice it. If not, you can try the simple method we teach at our workshops.

1. Sit comfortably. If you can, sit with one or both legs crossed. If not, you can sit on a chair.
2. Straighten your back and close your eyes.
3. Put the tip of your tongue behind your upper palate.
4. Inhale and exhale through your nose.
5. Relax and empty your mind.
6. You can silently speak to the sick parts of your body, "I'm sorry. Please forgive me. Thank you. I love you."
7. *Vipassana* meditation is even better.
8. During meditation, you may burp and pass gas. It's natural to shake and feel nausea, dizziness, chest tightness, energetic and blood flow changes, sudden changes in body temperature, soreness, numbness, swelling, and pain.
9. Your body might spontaneously move. It might feel frightening but stay positive and grateful to your body and nature.
10. *PaidaLajin* and meditation are complementary.
11. After practicing *PaidaLajin*, many meditators can now sit cross-legged—who could not do so before.
12. Meditation becomes easier over time.

19

DIETARY ADVICE AND ISSUES WITH COLD

I. Eat staple foods

The staple foods are the main things we eat, including rice, wheat, and other grains.

According to Chinese Medicine, staple foods are normally neutral, making them the least toxic to the human body. We can eat staple foods all year. Grains have been our main food since we became a farming civilization.

Meat, fruits, and vegetables are generally not neutral. They can be cold, cool, warm, or hot in nature. Eating too much can be harmful, so they can't be a staple food.

In other words, neutral food minimally interferes with the human body. It is the most suitable diet for us.

Herbal medicines are also hot or cold in nature, and they can be used to rebalance *yin-yang*. Chinese Medicine believes that "medication is more or less toxic." Do not take medicine unless it is absolutely necessary.

Modern science studies the chemical elements of food, medicine, and nutrients. It tends to focus on the parts, not the whole. Chinese Medicine is based on the theories of *qi* and *yin-yang*; it is holistic. *Qi* is a subtle vibration frequency. Each plant has a unique *qi* frequency. The traditional Chinese character 藥 (medicine) is composed of 艹 (grass, herbs) and 樂 (music.) Music is a combination of frequencies, and 藥 medicine is the music of medicinal herbs. Depending on their frequencies, food is neutral in nature, non-staple food is not neutral in nature (either cool or warm), and medicinal herbs are far from neutral in nature (either cold or hot.)

Everything in the universe has its own frequency, including matter, colors, and sounds. In the human body, the heart has a frequency (heartbeat), and every organ and cell has its own frequency. When these vibrate harmoniously as a whole, the human body is healthy and melodious—like a wonderful symphony.

Otherwise, the person is sick. There are "noises" amid the symphony. Herbs of different frequencies create interference waves. They strengthen or weaken cells, organs, and meridians: removing the excess and replenishing the deficiency. Ultimately, everything is regulated, harmony is restored, and *yin-yang* is balanced. This is how medicinal herbs and food work in the human body. Vibration frequency is both subtle and powerful. It is more accurate and comprehensive than biochemical substances.

Scientific study can lead to an incomplete understanding of food and medicine. Chemically synthetized drugs are usually removed from the market sooner or later because of side effects. However, in Chinese Medicine, the Theory of Homologous Food and Medicine has been practiced for several millennia. The efficacy of food and Chinese Medicine on health has been maintained throughout that time.

Many people refuse to eat staple foods for fear the starch will make them fat. In fact, the real cause of obesity is illness and blocked meridians.

In Chinese Medicine, nutrition and toxicity are relative, flexible concepts. According to the Theory of Homologous Food and Medicine, too little or too much of them is toxic, whereas a moderate amount is nutritious. When the foods and medicinal herbs are suitable for a person at a certain time, they are nutritious. Otherwise they are toxic. For instance, arsenic, whose chemical constituents are highly toxic, can effectively treat a certain cancer. In this sense, it is nutritious to the patient. By contrast, if you eat too much tasty, nutritious food, it is harmful to your health.

II. Eat less

Doctors, scientists, and health experts in the East and West have reached a rare consensus on the amount of food a person is supposed to eat: it is better to eat less—and it is even better to frequently fast.

Chinese Medicine believes eating less will reduce the energy needed for digestion. People who eat less have fewer desires and are more at peace. They will be healthy and energetic, and live longer. This is consistent with Taoism, Buddhism, and Confucianism. For millennia, Chinese people have personally experimented with this concept.

Initially, some Western scientists experimented on mice. They divided the mice into three groups, giving them excessive, moderate, and small portions of food. The mice who ate the most suffered from illness and died earliest. The group that ate the least was the healthiest and lived the longest. Subsequent experiments on humans produced similar results.

The extreme form of eating less is fasting. Mahatma Gandhi, Father of India, was a lifelong vegetarian who often fasted. Whenever he got sick, he would stop eating. His illness would be self-healed. It worked every time.

There is a saying in Chinese Medicine that, "A person can live a long life in spite of the illnesses he or she has." Indeed, some people born in poor health pay attention to dietary regulation and balance in life. They are able to enjoy longevity. Many people who are naturally strong exploit this advantage. They eat and drink too much, and then become very ill and die early.

American scientists once did an anatomical study on deceased people who lived over 100 years. Their findings proved the Chinese saying that many of those who enjoyed longevity had cancer, heart disease, and various other common diseases. But they maintained peace of mind and kept the *yin-yang* balance.

III. Become a vegetarian

Many people eat various meat products as their staple food. They eat little or no rice, wheat, or other grains. People love meat for nutrition or a variety of other reasons, especially the pleasure of eating meat—similar to smoking, drinking, and drug use. Many believe eating meat is an indispensable part of a happy life. But there are consequences.

Likewise, people become vegetarian for a variety of reasons: out of compassion, for better health, or because of environmental concerns. A vegetarian diet makes the meridians smoother, which is the best nourishment for the body.

Our physiological structure shows we are omnivorous; we can be either vegetarians or meat eaters. However, from the perspective of health preservation, vegetarian food is more suitable for us. It's easier to digest.

Carnivorous animals are born to be meat eaters—they have sharp teeth, short intestines for rapid excretion, and enough gastric acid to easily digest meat.

Herbivores have flatter teeth. Their intestines are long and winding, so it's hard to excrete waste.

Our teeth and intestines are similar to those of herbivores, and we can't produce much gastric acid to digest meat. Eating meat increases the workload of the spleen and stomach. Moreover, mass-produced meat is very toxic. Some girls start their periods too early, partly because of the hormones in the meat they eat. Chemical feeds make the animals grow fat and mature quickly. When people eat the meat, they become part of the vicious cycle. Early maturity leads to early aging and death.

The hospitals mirror the causes and effects of illness. If you go for an investigation there, you will find many are sick from overeating and eating meat.

I met an old couple once that both suffered from diabetes, hypertension, and hyperlipemia. They had a hard time walking due to pain, and they ate meat every day. I advised them to go vegetarian, or at least eat less meat and more grains, and practice *PaidaLajin* for three hours a day. Their pain and disease were gone. This is just one example.

Once, while chatting with a friend, I said, "Herbivores have more strength than carnivorous animals."

He countered, "Aren't the lions and tigers stronger?"

I replied, "They are strong, but their strength is mostly explosive force. It can't last long. That is why they hide for hours, waiting for a perfect opportunity to dash and catch their prey. The animals with the most stamina are herbivores, such as cattle, horses, donkeys, and elephants. Besides, carnivorous animals get their nutrition from eating herbivores, whose source is still vegetarian."

"Explosive force is also important for humans," he said.

I explained, "For a sprinter or a weightlifter, explosive force is indeed very important. But you are not an athlete. Isn't your sex life more important to you than sprinting and weight lifting? Which is more essential in your sex life—stamina or explosive force?"

On hearing this, my friend burst into laughter. And his wife laughed even harder.

So, why not try vegetarian food for your health, for our environment, out of compassion, or for religious reasons? If you can't be a vegan, it is good to mainly eat vegetarian food. At least it is good for your own health.

IV. Eat warm food and stay warm

We should eat warm food, because most diseases are cold induced.

We should eat food that's warmer than body temperature. If it's not as warm, your body has to work to warm it up, so your spleen can use the nutrients. Cold food leads to spleen, stomach, and intestinal problems.

We should also avoid food that is cool or cold in nature. According to Chinese Medicine, food can be cold, cool, neutral, warm, or hot.

If you eat a lot of food that is cold in nature (such as bitter gourd, green tea, or cool herbal tea), you can get sick—even if you warm up the temperature.

Many people with excessive internal fire like food and drink that is cool or cold in nature. But the cold is what caused the excessive internal fire in the first place. It blocks meridians, so toxins and waste can't be easily excreted through the urine, stool, and skin pores. As a result, acne, eczema, toothaches, itchiness, and other symptoms will crop up.

Excessive internal fire will disappear if you practice *PaidaLajin*, and drink ginger and jujube tea to boost your energy. Some people don't like to drink the tea; they even avoid the smell of it. The cold in their body is fighting against the heat of the tea. Normally, after *PaidaLajin*, they begin to enjoy it.

Many overweight people sweat a lot and love cold beverages. The real cause of obesity is too much cold; the heat is an illusion. Cold drinks lead to *qi* deficiency. When the *qi* can't be kept inside the body, the heat of *yang* easily evaporates. An overweight person is constantly sweating, because the body is too weak to keep the heat inside. Indeed, an obese person may feel hot—but is cold inside. The same is true with people who have acne.

Drinking cold beverages can, in the long run, contribute to coldness in the spleen and stomach. Undigested food remains in the body, since it can't be excreted. It accumulates in the form of fat and blood toxins. This especially leads to heart disease. Many obese people are unaware of their own heart disease. When slapped on their inner elbows, they experience a lot of pain and *sha*. These are indicators. When the skin there breaks, it's indicative of severe heart problems.

Many women suffer from the following cold-induced problems:

- Headaches
- Menstrual pain
- Irregular menstruation

- Cold hands and feet
- Weak, sore, and painful waists and knees
- Body weakness and fatigue

Apart from psychological pressure, most of these problems are caused by too much fruit, cold drinks, ice cream, and raw vegetables. People need more grains and other staple foods, and to spend more time in the sunshine. Even their eyes need some sunshine. If their eyes tear up, it is a detoxifying, healing reaction. The skin needs even more sun. Darker, itchy skin is also a detoxifying, healing reaction.

Ginger and Jujube Tea Recipe

- Cut ginger into slices
- Add a dozen or more red jujubes
- Boil in water for twenty to thirty minutes
- Add some brown sugar
- Please remember to drink it warm

OTHER ISSUES CAUSED BY COLD

Some women love fashion more than warmth. They wear clothes that expose their shoulders, waists, belly buttons, legs, and feet. Such clothing is very harmful to a woman's health. When a woman stays in an air-conditioned office wearing a skirt, stockings, and sandals, all her leg and feet meridians are exposed to the cold air. These include the Liver, Spleen, Stomach, Kidney, Gall Bladder, and Urinary Bladder Meridians. They lead up to the belly, uterus, and all internal organs. When all of these are cold, why wouldn't she be sick? In fact, a cold uterus causes infertility in many women.

It is very harmful for a woman in labor to stay in an air-conditioned room with a very low temperature. It is even worse for a woman undergoing a Cesarean section. The air-conditioning, surgery, and anesthesia during childbirth hurts her *qi* and blood. The post-childbirth infusions will inject even more cold into her weak body.

Infusions, antibiotics, and vaccinations make the mother and child colder, potentially causing a lifetime of pain and disease. Natural delivery is best. After childbirth, avoid air-conditioning, fruit, and infusions. Obesity, hemorrhoids, postpartum depression, and other symptoms are related to cold during prenatal and postpartum periods. Normally, a woman who undergoes a Cesarean section recovers more slowly than a woman who has a natural delivery. This is because the surgery and cold hurt the *qi* and blood more.

It is a natural law that things expand when hot and contract when cold. We humans are part of nature. Coldness leads to meridian restriction. In Chinese Medicine, cold and heat are respectively *yin* and *yang* in nature. A person's life from birth to death is a process of rising *yin* energy and falling *yang*. This is why people like to go to sunny places for holidays, and many move to warmer places after retirement. When we are more conscious of the hazards of cold, we will avoid these food and drinks. Zhang Zhongjing, Sage of Chinese Medicine, wrote "Discussion of Cold-Induced Disorders." Note that he didn't write about heat-induced disorders.

There are heat-induced diseases, but they are very rare—even in tropical regions. Heat stroke is one example. Luckily, not many people in developed countries work long hours under the scorching sun. When people spend time in a constant temperature—artificially created by air conditioning—they are isolated from nature. Their immunity declines. People in tropical areas are now suffering from more and more cold-induced problems, such as arthritis, diabetes, hypertension, heart disease, and lower back and leg pain. In some places (for instance, Hong Kong), the temperature in the subway, hotels, and shopping malls is kept at or below twenty degrees Celsius all year round. Just imagine how much pain and disease are man-made! It is the result of government policy. Why go against nature, waste so much energy, create disease, and pollute the environment?

In a word, to preserve good health:

- Stay warm and eat warm food
- Avoid cold food and drinks
- Reduce your reliance on air-conditioning

Of course, it's fun to occasionally have ice cream or drink a cold beer. But if we can replace cold beverages with warm ginger and jujube tea as a daily drink, there will be much fewer ill patients and health problems.

20

FREQUENTLY ASKED QUESTIONS

Paida looks like torture. Why would you beat yourself and other people?

Paida and *sha* look frightening. Getting used to the pain takes a while, and you aren't certain it will go away. Many people believe they are continuing to damage their body until they discover that *sha* and pain disappear if you continue slapping.

Many who practice *Paida* joke they have never been beaten so much, so hard, in their entire lives. Some of these people used to be doubters as well.

We learn to enjoy rhythm of *Paida*, and we learn to appreciate the healing that takes place after the pain disappears. We appreciate taking our health into our own hands. *Paida* becomes a normal part of our lives.

If you are open to the idea, research and try it yourself. After several rounds of *Paida*, your reactions will lessen, and you will become a much healthier person.

How does _Paida_ work?

The skin closely links to the meridian system, limbs, internal organs, and the nine orifices (eyes, ears, nostrils, mouth, urethra, and anus.)

Paida is an all-round activation of the slapped skin, the underlying muscles, bones, meridians, tendons, ligaments, blood vessels, nervous system, and all other systems of the body.

The slapped area automatically gathers more *qi* and blood. *Qi* propels blood flow. *Paida* improves *qi* and blood circulation. The enhanced *qi* acts as a cleaner—it automatically scans the entire body, identifying meridian blockages and removing them.

Paida boosts the power of the Heart and your confidence in self-healing.

From the perspective of Western Medicine, *Paida* is a proactive sabotage that stimulates the central nervous system (CNS) to repair damage, thus enhancing the body's self-repair capacity and immunity. This impacts:

- Energy
- Blood
- Various secretions
- The nervous, immune, and lymphatic systems

Is *Sha* Broken Blood Vessels?

No. People, even some TCM doctors, may be suspicious—or even scared—of *sha*. They assume *sha* is blood from ruptured blood vessels, and that it's dangerous. It isn't.

Our blood vessels behave somewhat like a rubber hose: when a hose is free of blockages, slapping or pressing it causes the water inside to flow to low-pressure areas. If there are no toxins blocking blood vessels during *Paida*, clean blood will flow from the slapped area to other areas. This explains why there is little to no *sha* in healthy body parts.

If you don't filter *sha* out of the body, it continues to stagnate and form harmful, pathogenic substances, such as:

- Fat
- Phlegm
- Masses
- Tumors
- Dampness

Blood vessel walls are a tight, mesh-like structure. Toxic waste makes the blood dense and highly viscous, substantially slowing down its flow. When you slap a stagnated area, a series of biochemical reactions takes place between toxins and *qi*.

Sha is very thick; some forms are almost solid. *Paida* exerts pressure on blood vessels, forcing the mesh openings to expand. *Sha* continues the biochemical fight with the boosted *qi*, and it's broken down into tiny particles.

Some particles go out through skin pores, like dust into the air. Others are excreted in sweat, tears, and nasal discharge. Most are excreted in urine and stool. Repeated slaps on the skin makes more *sha* cling to the walls.

Some people haven't been convinced. They've gone to the hospital for various tests, but they discover their blood vessels aren't broken. Other people have done the entire *Paida* process. They've taken pictures every step of the way, until all of the *sha* is gone.

Give it a try: *Paida* until *sha* appears. If you continue slapping the same area long and hard enough, *sha* will disappear, even if it takes over an hour.

In very rare cases, *Paida* causes capillaries under the skin to rupture. If your hand has sticky fluids or traces of blood on it, the skin and capillaries have indeed ruptured. This, however, is a great sign. Normal, healthy skin won't break during *Paida*. When capillaries rupture, the skin needs to break before it can heal (no destruction, no construction.) Old injuries, cold-dampness, and deeply buried toxins are being expelled. This is similar to bloodletting therapy, which is used by major ethnic groups around the world. In this case, *Paida* is killing two birds with one stone; you get the benefits of both *Paida* and bloodletting.

I have encountered many bleeding cases during *Paida* sessions. A man with severe heart problems had black *sha* on his inner elbow during his first *Paida* session. Blood seeped out from the *sha*, and he immediately felt his chest relax. His blood pressure dropped soon afterward.

In another man, after a few moments, the area along the Pericardium Meridian (on his inner elbow) turned purplish black. *Paida* quickly relieved the tightness in his chest. The palm he used for *Paida* was covered in blood. His chronic heart disease greatly improved, and his headaches, chest pain, and irregular heartbeat all disappeared.

I asked a strong practioner to *Paida* my shoulder with great force. By the end of the session, a large bloody blister had developed on his palm, where the Pericardium Meridian runs. His heart disease quickly improved, and the dark coloring on his face and lips faded.

For eczema, psoriasis, other skin diseases, and bites by toxic insects and animals, slap the areas until blood and sticky fluids are excreted. Slapping the skin until blood seeps out quickly reduces blood pressure in people with hypertension and heart disease. It also relieves headaches, chest tightness, and irregular heartbeats.

The skin will stop bleeding soon, scabs will form—and new, healthy skin will grow.

Cracks, water, or blood blisters might appear on the hands. They will subside and heal without any treatment.

After tough skin breaks, it will eventually be replaced by smoother, more delicate skin. Some people even experience systemic skin peeling—a free, natural skin resurfacing treatment!

Is *Sha* a Bruise?

No. Medical tests demonstrate there are no broken blood vessels during *sha*, except in the rare instances the skin breaks.

By contrast, bruises or injuries from a fight or accident are caused by sudden force. There is a lot of negative energy involved. There is excessive pain, and there might be scarring. Very often, the experience leaves emotional trauma long after it's over.

Does *Sha* Lead to Strokes or Heart Attacks?

No. Many people are puzzled by the disappearance of *sha* after *Paida*. Some doctors, who have never practiced *Paida*, imagine *sha* will re-enter blood circulation and lead to a stroke or a heart attack. This is not possible.

Detoxification through *PaidaLajin* isn't simply cleaning. *Qi* decomposes the toxic waste. The physical and chemical properties of the waste have been changed, so *sha* can only be excreted. This is the magic of our self-healing process.

Our skin is the largest detoxifying channel for *sha* because of countless pores. Each pore constantly breathes, just like the nostrils. The *yang* energy activated by *PaidaLajin* decomposes *sha* into tiny particles that are invisible to the naked eye. Because they are so small, they can escape through the pores. All other orifices, including our mouths, nostrils, eyes, ears, urethras, and anus are also detoxification channels. Burping, vomiting, sweating, nasal discharge, tears, earwax, farting, urine, and stool all convey detoxification. In short, excretions are always waste being removed from the body.

Sha is eliminated through these channels—it isn't reabsorbed. Without the biochemical reactions caused by *PaidaLajin*, these toxins will never be filtered out. They will continue to form pathogenic substances. During *PaidaLajin*, a person's sweat, urine, and stool will smell stronger than usual. It is normal to feel tired, because *sha* formation and removal consume energy.

According to Western Medicine, *sha* is 'poisoned blood' removed from blood vessels; it lies in the interstitial spaces under the skin. Interstitial blood is identified as an alien substance by phagocytes and lymphocytes, and they destroy and dispose of it. Phagocytes 'eat' harmful waste and lymphocytes attack toxins. When phagocytes and lymphocytes function normally, *sha* decomposes quickly. Regular *Paida* enhances the immune functions of these cells, helping the body to efficiently remove pathological substances.

Modern medical science has proven that removing harmful substances can enhance the function of the immune system, stimulate stem cell generation, and remove dying and dead skin cells—improving the body's capacity to cope with stress and repair damaged tissues.

Paida also serves as a DIY serum-antigen therapy, which makes the use of injections unnecessary.

Whether it be *Qi* Movement Theory and the *Yin-Yang* Interaction Theory in Chinese Medicine, or lymphatic or immune system theories in Western Medicine—we use our limited knowledge to decipher the unfathomable self-healing mechanism embedded in us. To truly uncover the secrets, you need to engage in the actual practice and experience it in your Heart.

Does *Lajin* Damage Tendons and Muscles?

No. You can adjust your practice to avoid injury.

Some people say their tendons have been stiff since childhood. This indicates that something is wrong with the liver, as the liver governs the tendons. These people should practice *Lajin* more than others.

If you don't experience pain, numbness, or swelling—no matter how long you practice *Lajin*—your bones are in place and your tendons are flexible. *Qi* and blood can flow naturally, and you don't need to practice *Lajin* any longer.

What is the Best Time of Day to Practice *PaidaLajin*?

As we often say, "Rome is not built in a day."

Illnesses are built up over time; likewise, it takes time to heal them. A person can get sick at any time of a day and any day of a year; *PaidaLajin* can be practiced at any moment of a day and in any season of a year.

Generally speaking, it is best to practice *PaidaLajin* in the morning when *yang* is rising. If you have a rich knowledge of Chinese Medicine and flexibility in your schedule, you can follow the midnight-midday ebb flow of *qi* in the meridian system. But people have different rhythms in life and work, and they can't all practice *PaidaLajin* at a certain time. As the saying goes, "Why choose the best time? Now is the time."

Now is the time for *PaidaLajin*.

Don't forget the importance of your mindset. With genuine gratitude and repentance in the Heart, the healing effect will be even greater. Illness originates in the Heart—and the cure also comes from the Heart.

Can You Practice *PaidaLajin* in Winter—The Season of Preserving Energy?

Yes. According to Chinese Medicine, winter is the season when we are supposed to preserve our energy.

People with some knowledge of Chinese Medicine often ask, "Can *PaidaLajin* be practiced in winter?" The underlying assumption is we should focus only on preserving energy and replenishing deficiencies in winter. Another common question is, "Which of the four seasons is the best time to practice *PaidaLajin*?"

PaidaLajin can be practiced in all four seasons, and at any time of the day. You can get sick at any time. Therefore, disease treatment can happen at any time. We should preserve good energy in the winter—not toxic waste. *PaidaLajin* removes the excesses and replenishes the deficiencies It is automatically regulated within the body.

If you are 100% healthy, you can follow the seasonal health-keeping regime. But such people are very rare. If you have poor health, it means you either have current illnesses, latent illnesses, or both. The top priority is curing disease by dredging the meridians. If you get sick in winter, do you wait until the next spring to receive treatment? Do you wait until a minor illness worsens to a grave problem?

Why should we heal diseases in certain hours and seasons, but not in others?

Indeed, Chinese Medicine advocates the preservation of energy in winter.

However, what should be preserved in winter are the "top-quality fruits" we gather in the autumn. When a person is sick, in addition to the visible tumors, lumps, and phlegm, there can be invisible cold and toxic *qi* in the meridian system, cells, organs, bones, and blood. Are we expected to preserve the waste, toxins, and negative energy in the body?

More importantly, *PaidaLajin* is more than simple detoxification. It turns toxins into nutrients. It enhances positive energy, while getting rid of negative energy. This process of transformation serves the purpose of absorbing nutrition. What better way to preserve energy?

Without detoxification, elimination of cold-dampness, and the conversion of waste into nutrients, what is preserved in winter could be a pile of garbage and negative energy.

This transformation process makes room for nutrition and positive energy. With abundant positive energy, the negative energy will recede, and *yin-yang* balances. A well-balanced person is a healthy person. Boost your positive energy first—and then work to conserve it.

Seen from another perspective, winter is a cold season, but also a festive and feasting season. The mortality rates can be higher than usual. Acute diseases occur more frequently, particularly strokes, hypertension, heart attacks, and gastrointestinal disorders. Hospitals are often overcrowded. This is when there is a greater need for *PaidaLajin*. It helps people and also lessens the pressure on hospitals.

When *PaidaLajin* is practiced conscientiously in spring, summer, and autumn as well, we will all enjoy better health in winter.

According to Chinese Medicine, similar to the four seasons in a year, there are also 'four seasons' in a twenty-four-hour day.

Our first *PaidaLajin* workshop was held in the winter of 2010 in Beijing. You can draw your own conclusion from the statistics in the book on a second Beijing workshop that year.

Is *PaidaLajin* Suitable for the Elderly, Gravely Ill Patients, and People with Weak Qi?

Yes. Typically, gravely ill patients and elderly people suffer *qi* and blood deficiency.

Thousands of examples of clinical evidence show that of all the people practicing *PaidaLajin*, whether at home or in a workshop, the people most likely to show strong results are elderly, gravely ill, and deficient in *qi* and blood. Some are so deficient the body can't absorb much nutrition. This can't be remedied immediately; it will take time and work. When the supply channels in the body are blocked, the nutrition and drugs can't reach their destination. When the road is narrow, or when there is a traffic accident, putting more vehicles on the road does not help. The first task is to clear the road.

It has been proven in front-line scientific research that bones, joints, skin, muscles, and tendons are not only kinematic systems—they are the largest human endocrine system. Practicing *PaidaLajin* clears meridians, blood vessels, lymphatic vessels, the nervous system, and other bodily systems, optimizing blood and organ function. This not only enhances the immune system; it turns waste into treasure.

This is clearly explained in Chinese Medicine. *PaidaLajin*, aided by food therapy such as ginger and jujube tea, replenishes *yang*, which enhances circulation. Smoothly flowing meridians enhance *yang*, which acts as an anti-virus mechanism to remove viruses, excess fat, cancer cells, and tumors. Otherwise, nourishment entering the body may spur the growth of disease, since all of those dysfunctional conditions use nutrition to grow as well.

While practicing *PaidaLajin*, drink ginger and jujube tea, then move on to rice, bread, congee, noodles, and other staple foods. Choose simple, natural foods that are easy to digest. Chinese people have eaten these foods for millennia, and they have proven to be the best choices for replenishing *qi* and blood. Avoid taking drugs, and eating processed or canned foods. If you are very weak, take a break.

Can *PaidaLajin* Kill Bacteria and Cancer?

Not directly, but it balances bacteria and stops the growth of cancer.

Antibiotics are used to kill bacteria. However, resistant varieties continue to develop. In response, more powerful antibiotics are produced and prescribed to destroy these new varieties.

Humans and bacteria are dragged into a never-ending, vicious cycle.

Similarly, in the face of cancer, the mode of treatment is to kill cells with chemotherapy and remove tumors with surgery. When antibiotics, surgery, and chemotherapy are used to kill cells and tumors, the human body is treated as a lifeless machine without a soul. These treatments get rid of the "problems", while overlooking the causes. The unintended consequence of such therapeutic principles and treatments: they cover up the problems instead of uprooting them.

In Chinese Medicine, there is no such notion of destroying bacteria and cancer cells. Why kill them? Chinese Medicine emphasizes balance and harmony.

Bacteria are everywhere. You can find numerous bacteria in the air, water, plants, animals, a person's mouth, nostrils, and internal organs. They're in wine, butter, cheese, vinegar, and soy sauce. It is impossible to kill all bacteria. What humans can do is to maintain a balance between beneficial and harmful bacteria. Good balance contributes to good health. As long as *qi* and blood flow smoothly, there is a natural balance. *Yin-yang* equilibrium addresses these two different kinds of bacteria.

Similarly, in Chinese Medicine, you cure cancer by changing the environment of the body. Blocked meridians create an environment conducive to the growth of cancer cells. There is an old saying: "Running water is never stale, and a door-hinge in use is never worm-eaten." Chinese Medicine does not simply cut, kill, or eradicate. Cold, phlegm, dampness, stagnations, and toxins melt away, and pathogenic organisms either change their nature or are excreted.

Cupping, massage, acupuncture, moxibustion, Chinese herbal medicine, and other therapies all dredge meridians. These therapies are mostly reliant on professionals, unlike *PaidaLajin*.

Tumors and masses are *yin* in nature. As long as there is enough *yang* energy, the body is warmed up. Cancer cells can no longer exist in the changed environment.

In winter, ice blocks may be hard as stones. When spring comes and *yang* rises, they melt into water. As the temperature continues to rise, water evaporates and clouds are formed. When clouds up in the air meet low temperatures (*yin* energy), rain falls. Ancient Chinese described the natural phenomena as: "Gathering to form a tangible substance and evaporating into the air."

The crucial factor is the temperature. The birth and death of cancer cells follow the same law. In Chinese Medicine, the verb Hua (化; *pinyin: huà*) is often used, which means "to change, to convert, to dissolve." For instance, to hua phlegm, dampness and stagnation; to hua toxins into medicine, enemies into friends, and war into peace.

PaidaLajin does not target them directly. It simply starts the engine of a car with a key. That is all—and that is enough.

Will *PaidaLajin* Spread Bacteria and Cancer Cells?

No. *PaidaLajin* does not sweep cancer cells and pathogenic bacteria from one part of the body to another like garbage.

PaidaLajin may appear to be simple exercises, but—in addition to tuning the vibration frequencies of all cells and organs in the body—*PaidaLajin* enhances the subtlest *qi*, causing physical, biochemical, and psychological changes.

Cancer cells and pathogenic bacteria don't grow out of toxins. An unbalanced body is favorable for the growth of cancer cells and unhealthy bacteria, and inhibits the growth of healthy cells—including stem cells—and beneficial bacteria. Many factors contribute to the overgrowth of cancer cells and pathogenic bacteria, but ultimately stagnation of *qi* and blood is responsible—similar to mosquitoes and other insects gathering around dirty water. Removing energetic blockages so "running water does not get stale" results in organic, holistic self-healing.

"Where Should I Slap to Heal (Fill in the Blank)?"

This is the most frequently asked question.

It reveals a mode of thinking typical in modern medicine: get rid of the symptoms instead of the cause.

This thinking is linear and compartmentalized, rather than holistic and systematic.

As a reminder, all diseases are complex diseases based on meridian blockages.

Even a mild cold, cough, or fever indicates immune system disorders. Chronic diseases are a combination of many things—in other words, the blockages of multiple meridians.

Systematically practice *PaidaLajin* in a systematic manner. Don't just slap a certain region for the sake of curing a particular symptom unless it's an emergency.

Huang Di Nei Jing and *The Tao Te Ching* provide theoretical guidelines for *PaidaLajin*. *Yin-yang* interactions, the meridian system, and action through inaction, stated in the two classics are indispensable for establishing an understanding of *PaidaLajin*.

Beginners can read the "Journey to Self-Healing" serials, in Chinese or English, on our websites. Hardback and paperback Chinese editions titled *Journey to Cure* were published in Taiwan and on the Chinese mainland. You can get a glimpse into Chinese Medicine and Western Medicine and their respective historical and cultural background. You will gain background knowledge in Chinese Medicine.

Disease names can be quite misleading, although they can also be useful for communication.

Descriptions in different parts of this book may overlap and seem repetitive, but we need to emphasize here: all illness is complex and different diseases can manifest the same symptoms.

The nature of a disease is *yin-yang* imbalance caused by meridian blockages. The most essential task is unblocking the clogged meridians. Temporary exacerbation of certain symptoms during this process is a good thing, which we call "healing reactions"—the intertwining danger of a seeming decline in health offers an opportunity for thorough healing.

We receive steady requests asking us to disclose the secret of *PaidaLajin* for healing certain illnesses. But people will invariably find that the so-called secret formula is simple common sense. There is no secret at all. "The greatest way is the simplest."

How long can people live?

Theoretically, everyone can live to be 120 years old. According to Sun Simiao, the king of Chinese Medicine during the Tang Dynasty—who lived to be over one hundred years old: "Human life is of paramount importance, more precious than a thousand pieces of gold."

What roles does the meridian system play?

The meridian system is the cradle of vitality, the origin of the onset of illnesses, the nest of the progress of the illnesses—and the key to curing a patient.

Why should I balance the way I use my body?

1. Overusing your eyes hurts your blood.
2. Reclining too long restricts *qi*.
3. Sitting too much is bad for your muscles.
4. Standing too long can damage your bones.
5. Excessive walking or running harms jin (your tendons and ligaments.)

Why should I work to manage my emotions?

Emotions disturb the circulation in various organs:

Anger—Liver

Fear—Kidneys

Sadness—Lungs

Over-thinking—Spleen
Overjoy—Heart

Emotions and temperature can also affect the flow and speed of *qi*.

Anger—speeds it up
Overjoy—slows it down
Anxiety—lowers it
Cold—diminishes it
Heat—disperses it
Fear—disorients it
Hard work—exhausts it
Overthinking—freezes it

What is healthy living?

In ancient times, people who knew The Tao balanced *ying* and *yang*, preserved their health, practiced restraint when eating and drinking, kept regular hours, and rested enough. They were healthy throughout their natural lifespans, around 100 years of age.

What is unhealthy living?

Today's people drink liquor like water, practice irresponsible sex, pursue desires the way they should requirements, and burn themselves out seeking pleasure. It disrupts their bodies, depleting vital energy and their essence by the time they're fifty.

What should I do when I'm sick?

The first priority is to nurse the Heart. Then apply external treatment and dietary therapies. Use medication as the last resort.

What is the best kind of doctor?

- A superior healer treats future illnesses.
- An average healer treats impending illness.
- A poor doctor only treats someone who is already ill.

The best doctor clears away possible problems long before their onset. Now, you can practice *PaidaLajin*—and be a superior doctor for yourself.

How can I stay healthy?

If there's positive *qi* inside us, it protects us from external damaging forces.

Clear yourself of greed and excessive thinking to maintain your positive *qi*. Disease can't live in that kind of environment.

Why are the spleen and kidneys essential to health and longevity?

The spleen and the kidneys are directly related to *qi*. Almost all illnesses are associated with deficient energy in these organs.

Chinese Medicine advocates nourishing the spleen, stomach, and kidneys to maintain good health and slow down aging. Prenatal *qi* is stored in the kidneys, and the spleen absorbs nutrition from the food we eat. A person with abundant kidney energy is energetic. They have healthy hair and bones, good hearing and eyesight, and healthy sexual and reproductive functions. A person with deficient kidney energy is listless and may not have a healthy sex life.

Men are more afraid of kidney deficiency than women. Various kidney drug advertisements encourage men to "be strong." They give the impression that these drugs and supplements will boost sexuality. Also, a man with deficient kidney energy tends to have prostate disorders.

In fact, women can suffer more from severe kidney deficiency than men. A woman with deficient kidney energy tends to have gynecological disorders. Deficiency is caused by overuse and early aging. We need to know and enhance the kidney's functions.

The kidneys and the urinary bladder are a pair; they thrive or wither together. Nourishing one nourishes the other. When stretching on a *Lajin* bench, the Urinary Bladder Meridian hurts the most—and kidney energy soars as a result.

In addition to boosting the kidneys, we need to nourish the spleen and stomach with a balanced diet. The body relies on prenatal *qi* to warm up and digest food. They are interdependent.

Many people assume digestion occurs in the stomach, but the spleen and stomach work together to absorb and transport nutrition. It's similar to the way the kidneys and the urinary bladder govern the flow of liquids together.

When your stomach and spleen don't cooperate with each other, your digestion and sleep are impacted. In addition to diet, you must also get sufficient rest.

What damages the spleen and stomach?

According to the Five Elements Theory in Chinese Medicine, the spleen has the properties of earth, while the kidney holds the properties of water. The spleen limits the kidneys. When your spleen is sick, it damages your kidney energy as well, leading to further illness.

According to *Huang Di Nei Jing*, the spleen and stomach are responsible for food intake, as well as the absorption, conversion, and distribution of nutrients. In Chinese Medicine, they encompass the entire digestive system. According to the Five Elements Theory, the Spleen—with its properties of earth in the center—nourishes every organ and cell in the body. By impacting the four elements of wood (liver), fire (heart), metal (lung), and water (kidneys), there are connections in all directions.

The stomach receives the food we eat, grinds it into small particles, and warms it up. The spleen absorbs various nutrients from these particles, converts them into what the body needs, and transports the right amount of nutrition to wherever it is needed.

A spleen-stomach imbalance will impact the absorption, conversion, and distribution of nutrients. It also causes problems with the discharge of waste and toxins. The internal organs will lack nourishment, weakening their function. Phlegm and stagnant blood will accumulate.

This imbalance ultimately creates a decline in health—or possibly even death.

I often hear people ask vegetarians and those who eat less food, "Do you get enough nutrition? Will you get sick?" If you go to the hospital and conduct a survey, you will find that problems with the heart, liver, stomach, and kidneys are associated with too much food intake. Which of these diseases are caused by hunger? What about obesity? Well, you know the answer.

Why are so many people overweight? Why do so many of us suffer from spleen and stomach problems? The reason is because we eat so much that full digestion is not possible. Many people want to lose weight, but they ignore the root cause and assume they can get rid of extra fat like cutting hair. This isn't a good system.

Huang Di Nei Jing states that a healthy person possesses adequate vitality. The vitality is converted from the kidney energy. Both prenatal and postnatal influences determine whether there is abundant vital energy. *Compendium of Materia Medica* says, "The spleen nourishes all organs and cells in the body. When a person's spleen is healthy, the heart, liver, lungs, and kidneys will be functioning normally, evil energies will go away, and he or she will have no illnesses."

Eating nutritious food is not enough. When food enters the body, the spleen and stomach have to bear a huge workload. The stomach, which functions well when it is 70% full, is often stuffed with food till 170% full. The poor spleen and stomach overwork every day, even when we're asleep. How could we not get sick?

How should I fast?

Fasting means not eating for a set amount of time.

Fasting enables the spleen and stomach to rest. Since ancient times, people have developed various methods of fasting. However, many are too complex and mysterious. What we teach is very simple; you don't need to prepare. As long as you feel you are ready, you can fast for three to seven days. When the Heart decides to fast, all the internal organs will collaborate to make it happen. During the fasting period, you can drink warm water or ginger and jujube tea. This is intermittent fasting. In strict fasting, intake of water is also avoided.

In our seven-day workshop, there is a three-day fasting period. Most people don't feel hungry. Many participants feel great at the end of the period and choose to fast for a few more days. In addition, we spend eight hours a day doing *Paida*, *Lajin*, meditation, Zen jogging, wall hitting, waist swirling, and *tie qiang gong* exercises. The energy boosted through these activities burns up waste and pathogens, converting them into natural medicine. It is like generating power from garbage. This is one reason why people don't feel hungry when fasting. *PaidaLajin* during fasting helps participants to detoxify, slim down, self-heal diseases, and move energy through their bodies.

Some people experience various healing reactions during fasting, including fatigue, nausea, vomiting, and dizziness. These are good reactions. It is a better to eject vomit of various colors. Toxins and wastes in the lower part of the body can be easily excreted through urine and stool. Toxins in the upper body are trapped in the lungs, spleen, stomach, esophagus, and respiratory tract. These can't be discharged easily. Vomiting during fasting and *PaidaLajin* is one of the best ways to get rid of them.

If you do not want to fast, eating less is an option.

People with hypoglycemia (low blood sugar), brain ischemia, or stomach problems eat whenever they feel hungry, and they take candy wherever they go. These people, more so than others, should fast. They not only have stomach problems, but heart disease as well—though they might not be aware of it yet. When they feel dizzy and hungry as a result of ischemia and hypoglycemia, *Paida* their inner elbows and *Neiguan* Acupoints. Many stomach problems and hypoglycemic syndromes are healed by *PaidaLajin*, since heart disease is behind these superficial symptoms.

Why should I drink less water?

This is contrary to the popular belief that you should drink lots of water to detoxify. Chinese Medicine advocates only drinking water when you are thirsty—and drinking it at room temperature.

It is true that a large proportion of the human body is water, and that water can help detoxify the body. However, the pre-condition is smoothly flowing meridians. *Qi* sustains the circulation of both water and blood. We drink water, and discharge urine and sweat. This shows that *qi*'s nature changes. In essence, it is *qi*—not water—that helps with detoxification. *Qi* takes water to all internal organs and cells; and it is *qi* that determines where the water flows, how much is retained in the blood and bodily fluids, and how much is excreted. So, meridian blockages change the flow of water as well. A dead person has no *qi*, and water poured into the dead body does not flow. It won't be changed into urine or sweat.

Turning water into urine takes energy, so drinking less water saves energy. If you drink gallons of water every day, in the long run you could suffer heart, kidney, and urinary bladder diseases. Other organs might malfunction as well.

Moreover, water is *yin* in nature. Icy cold water is even worse. When the sun is rising in the morning, the *yang* in your body is also rising. Don't drink a lot of water in the morning when *yang* is rising, especially cool or cold water. *Yang* will cool down before it has a chance to rise. According to Chinese Medicine, the Heart has the properties of fire, and many people give themselves heart disease when they put out this fire.

The biggest characteristic of heart disease is that it's deeply hidden. Normally it can't be detected during a medical checkup unless you are dying. Sometimes it isn't even detected when a person with a heart attack is sent to the hospital. Some people die in the hospital on the day of the checkup, but the report indicates nothing was wrong with their heart.

How do you diagnose whether a person with the habit of drinking cool water has heart disease or not? *Paida* the inner elbows. If there is pain and *sha*, then he or she has heart disease. Pain is a more accurate indicator than *sha*. A person with a healthy heart won't feel much pain there.

Why do some people often feel thirsty?

Because they are sick; their meridians are blocked. Normally, multiple meridians are blocked. Almost all diabetic patients have heart disease, and they are always thirsty. When a healthy person feels thirsty, he or she drinks some water and the thirst is gone. But a patient who constantly drinks can still feel thirsty if water doesn't move through all of their meridians. The more blockages, the more a person tends to drink. It's a vicious cycle.

Some people suffer from edema: including swelling of the face, eyes, legs, feet—or even their entire body. This is due to drinking too much water, which leads to malfunctioning of the kidneys and urinary bladder. To relieve edema, stretch on a *Lajin* bench, *Paida* the universal regions (elbows, knees, hands and feet), and then slap all along the four limbs. The edema will disappear.

A pregnant woman had systemic edema but avoided medicine for the sake of her baby. She slapped her limbs for a whole day, a lot of *sha* came out, and the edema cleared up. Three days later, she gave birth to a healthy baby.

I often go for a few days without drinking water, but I don't feel thirsty. There is enough water in the air and my food to meet my needs. It is more so in humid regions—you don't have to drink much water, because your skin can breathe. But if I dine out at a restaurant, I will feel very thirsty, due to MSG, salt, and other chemical seasonings. It is best to avoid them and eat natural foods.

There is a health expert who promotes a dietary therapy that separates food and water. This is based on the interactions of *yin-yang* and the Five Elements in Chinese Medicine.

Why is swimming too often bad for me?

Your body absorbs cold-dampness through your pores when you're in a swimming pool if the water is too cold. If you're over thirty, your *yang* is already declining. It's OK to swim occasionally, but it's not a good daily exercise.

Why shouldn't I take supplements?

All medicines, including supplements, have side effects since they aren't neutral in nature. Even if the diagnosis is correct, there might be issues. Medical institutions have studied them and drawn similar conclusions—over-supplementation induces disease.

Sometimes, supplements can be even more dangerous than prescribed medicine. They can be readily purchased and are widely used. Many supplements industrially produced.

Ask yourself:

1. How do I know these nutrients are exactly what my body needs?
2. How do I know if I can absorb these nutrients?
3. Can my body move the supplements everywhere it needs them?

When these nutrients enter the human body, they can be easily 'eaten' by pathogenic life forms. Instead of nourishing your health, they can potentially fuel the diseases! Tumors, cancer, sputum, bacteria, and inflamed tissue all need food as well.

I have often asked doctors and nutrition experts:

1. Are you sure the medicine and nutrition will reach the designated locations in the body?
2. How can you be sure?
3. How can you prevent medication and supplements from damaging healthy cells?

Up until now, no one has been able to answer these simple questions.

Return the job of diagnosis and healing to the Universal Life Force.

Although supplements are generally less toxic than drugs, long-term use can be poisonous. Some people take vitamins for decades, and they're still deficient in them. Even worse, many people who take calcium pills form kidney stones.

Many elderly people with leg pain are diagnosed with calcium deficiency and degenerative, irreversible diseases. However, after taking prescriptions and calcium for years, their symptoms haven't improved—some are even worse. When they stop taking these drugs and supplements and practice *PaidaLajin* instead, checkup result shows no calcium deficiency.

Why do both men and women suffer from kidney deficiency?

Chinese and Western Medicine agree the kidneys have urinary and reproductive functions.

According to Western Medicine, they are mainly the urinary organs, in charge of secreting and metabolizing fluids. Problems with the kidneys include nephropyelitis, glomerulonephritis (GN), kidney stones, and renal failure. They are also involved in nervous, endocrine, and respiratory functions, as well as energy metabolism. That's why both men and women tend to suffer from kidney deficiency.

In Chinese Medicine, the Kidney includes the physical kidneys, but they're also related to hair, ears, bones, teeth, and energy levels. They store prenatal *qi*, provide energy for birth and growth, and assist in the functioning of internal organs.

Why does kidney deficiency induce mood swings in women?

Nurse the Heart, first and foremost.

The Heart has the properties of fire, and the Kidney has the properties of water. A person suffers mood swings when the Heart and Kidney energies are discordant, meaning fire and water are unbalanced. With enough Kidney water, excessive Heart fire can be put out. Uncontrolled Heart fire flares up to the brain. This causes mood swings, overthinking, and insomnia.

A woman's kidney energy reaches its peak at twenty-eight. Then it begins to decline. Even women who don't have disorders will begin to see symptoms of kidney deficiency.

Female Kidney Deficiency:

- Insomnia
- Irritation
- Anxiety
- Suspicion
- Mood swings
- Hair loss
- Low libido
- Poor memory
- Impaired concentration
- Irregular menstruation
- Cold hands and feet

In a word, women feel uncomfortable all over. They lack energy, or it is out of control.

When a woman with kidney deficiency experiences the tug-of-water between Heart fire and kidney water, her body is turned into a battlefield. This creates mood swings—leading to yet another vicious cycle.

In addition to nursing the Heart, find ways to increase kidney water to put out the fire.

How can I boost my kidney energy?

Kidney deficiency is an inevitable part of a person's life cycle. As we get older, the function of our internal organs will weaken. The question is: how can we slow it down?

The right way to boost kidney energy is to eat and exercise properly. Follow our advice on eating and drinking, and waist swirling, *tie qiang gong*, and breathing exercises.

How can I get rid of chronic fatigue syndrome (CFS)?

Please reference the section on CFS in the "Steps for Specific Disorders" section.

What training do workshop coaches do?

A qualified coach must participate in a workshop at least ten times. They have successfully healed themselves. Every workshop has different cases, energies, and healing reactions. Coaches learn to be prepared in their Hearts to remain calm and soothe frightened participants.

Is *PaidaLajin* really free?

PaidaLajin greatly improves health and lowers medical spending.

According to surveys, almost 80% of workshop participants no longer need medication, and they're healthier than when they took the medicine.

Many people wish the workshops were free. Countless people have healed themselves without the workshop—without spending a penny. We are devoted to our blogs, Weibo, Wechat, Chinese, and English websites. They will teach you to heal yourself for free. It's not optimal, but you can practice *Lajin* for free, without a bench. You can also share a bench with others. You can make your own ginger and jujube tea for less money. It's still much cheaper than regular prescriptions and visits to the doctor.

Why aren't the workshops free?

Even though you can learn for free, please note that these offerings cost our organization. This leaves us with only one option—to conduct workshops like a business. We also sell *Lajin* benches and *Paida* sticks.

Hopefully the day will come when we do not need to worry about feeding our families or finding funds to travel. Then we will offer workshops for free.

Why do you address specific disorders if *PaidaLajin* must be applied to the entire body?

PaidaLajin should become a way to maintain health and prevent illness, and not a method for curing diseases. However, in today's world, people are most interested in disease treatment, so we promote *PaidaLajin* that way. It can heal all kinds of diseases, but it is not a guarantee.

We hope people will learn to be proactive and address their meridians before they are ill.

Do I need to learn about Chinese Medicine before practicing *PaidaLajin*?

No. Numerous people across the world without knowledge of Chinese Medicine are practicing and benefiting from *PaidaLajin*.

Of course, if you know some basics about Chinese Medicine and the meridian system, it helps you to better understand *PaidaLajin*. But many Western doctors and naturopaths can explain it from other perspectives as well.

Patting and stretching have always been natural, human movements. Clapping your hands, patting certain body parts, and stretching in various postures have long been practiced in many cultures as part of physical exercise and healing.

How can I learn *PaidaLajin* well?

There are now videos, *PaidaLajin* self-healing books, and websites in multiple languages. You can read and watch video tutorials to learn the philosophy, concepts, and techniques. You will also find links to relevant scientific reports and testimonials. You can probably find *PaidaLajin* self-healers—and those interested in learning more—in your family, community, city, or country.

I can't attend a workshop right now. Will that impact my recovery?

Attending a workshop is the best way to learn through experience. We teach and experience self-help *Paida* and mutual *Paida*, how to nurse the Heart, and how to deal with acute symptoms and healing reactions. We also teach fasting, meditation, Zen jogging, wall hitting, waist swirling, and tie qiang gong exercises. You get to bond with other people and interact with coaches. These are all aimed at empowering participants to self-heal.

However, many people have self-healed on their own. Then they write to us to share their self-healing experience. So can you. Persist in *PaidaLajin* and you will gradually recover. But it might take longer.

Are there video tutorials for *PaidaLajin*?

Yes. You can watch videos of *Paida*, *Lajin*, wall hitting, waist swirling, tie qiang gong, documentaries, testimonials, and interviews on the video section of our English website: http://www.*paidalajin*.com/en/home. You can also search for *Paida*, *Lajin*, and *PaidaLajin* on YouTube. DVD tutorials with Chinese and English subtitles are available at our Chinese online store.

Which of the *Lajin* postures is most suitable for me?

Of the seven *Lajin* postures we have recommended, *Lajin* in Reclining Posture (best on a *Lajin* bench) delivers the most comprehensive effects.

You can practice it to prevent and self-heal almost every meridian.

For other postures, choose according to your specific condition. If you have shoulder problems, you can practice *Lajin* in Standing Posture. For eye and neck problems, practice Neck *Lajin*, and sleep on a hard surface without a pillow. Do Standing on a Board *Lajin* for feet and leg problems. If you have difficulty squatting down, practice *Lajin* in Squatting Posture. *Lajin* in Y-Shaped Posture is the best for menstrual, liver, spleen, and kidney issues.

How can I get a *Lajin* bench?

You can buy one from us or one of our worldwide contacts (listed on the "service" section of our English website.) You can make your own *Lajin* bench by attaching a long pole to your bed, desk, or coffee table. This is only makeshift though. The bench is safer and more effective. The following dimensions are for your reference, but you can adjust them for your needs.

Length: 47 in. Width: 22 in. Height 22 in.

Pole length 67 in. Pole width: 3 in. Pole thickness: 1.2 in.

If possible, use sandbags or other weights on the legs when stretching on the bench.

Does *PaidaLajin* have side effects?

No. For a while, you experience healing reactions, but they aren't permanent. However, there are "by-products" people welcome: losing weight, getting taller, improving their figure, having better skin, increasing sexual function, and having more hair growth with a healthier color. Most importantly, you will get sick less often.

Is it OK to *Paida* your head?

Of course! At our workshop, we spend over an hour each morning slapping our heads and faces, including the top, left, right, front, and back sides of our heads. We also address our necks, foreheads, cheeks, eyes, ears, and mouths. Start lightly and increase the intensity as you adjust.

Regular *Paida* on these areas improves the health of the eyes and ears. It is particularly good for Alzheimer's patients. It lifts our spirits, prevents strokes and hair loss, and preserves and improves our hair and facial color. Insomnia, migraines, and other related illness will also gradually heal. People with baldness or bald patches often grow hair again with head *Paida*.

Can I get rid of acne?

Yes. Many people have removed acne and dark spots by doing *Paida* on their faces.

It may appear acne is a result of too much internal fire (inflammation.) In fact, it is caused by too much cold that can't be released due to meridian blockages.

You can slap your inner elbows, *Dazhui* Acupoints, chest, back, spine, and the back of your legs along the Urinary Bladder Meridians. Do *Lajin* on a bench. Avoid cold water and beverages. Eat less meat, fruits, and raw vegetables—all are cold in nature.

Can I *Paida* my breasts?

Yes. Nine main meridians go through the breasts. It helps with breast hyperplasia and breast cancer, as well as depression, heart disease, hypothyroidism, hyperthyroidism, ovarian cysts, and uterine fibroids. In addition, it contributes to natural breast enhancement and overall beauty.

Can I slap my belly?

Yes. Your belly is linked to your internal organs. There are many important acupoints on and around the belly button. Slapping the entire belly helps to relieve diabetes, hypertension, prostate disorders, and gynecological disorders. It's also good for heart, liver, kidney, stomach, and intestinal problems. It is a natural way to lose weight.

For a pregnant woman, please do not slap on the belly. It is OK to *Paida* other body parts.

Can I slap my hips and buttocks?

Yes. Many people sit a lot, so the buttocks bear a lot of the body's weight. Waste and toxins accumulate there. The Urinary Bladder Meridian (one of the biggest detoxification channels in the body), the Gall Bladder Meridian, and other important meridians run through the buttocks. Meridian blockages here can lead to obesity, diabetes, hypertension, heart disease, lower back pain, prostate disorders, gynecological disorders, stomach, intestinal, and reproductive problems. When you slap your hips, toxic waste can be expelled as colorful *sha*.

Can I slap scars?

Yes. You can slap on scars as a result of burns, scalds, surgery, or other injuries. It will help to further repair the damage, and it gets rid of cold and toxic waste. Do not slap on open wounds though.

Can I slap varicose veins?

Yes. Many people have protruding veins. Varicose veins are not a minor problem you should ignore. They not only impact the area of the veins, but also blood flow back to the heart, which impacts the entire body.

Paida the universal regions first (elbows, knees, hands and feet) to enable energy and blood flow. Then *Paida* directly at and around the varicose veins. Start with soft *Paida* and gradually slap harder. Normally, varicose veins can stand heavy *Paida*. There is no need to panic if they bleed a little. The protruding veins will typically flatten after thirty to sixty minutes. In severe cases, you will need to *Paida* for additional rounds.

Can I practice *PaidaLajin* during my period?

Yes. It is even more effective at this time. Many women experience pain and mood swings before and during their period. *PaidaLajin* helps relieve the pain, and it brings inner peace and smoothness of menstrual discharge. *Paida* the belly and along the inner side of each leg. *Lajin* in Y-Shaped Posture is particularly effective. Stay warm and drink ginger and jujube tea.

Can pregnant women practice *PaidaLajin*?

Yes. A pregnant woman can practice *PaidaLajin* during her entire period of pregnancy. It helps with edema, insomnia, nausea, vomiting, back pain, and waist pain. It also improves mood and flexibility, which enhances the health of the mother and the baby. It contributes to natural childbirth. DO NOT *Paida* the belly, though.

Can a woman practice *PaidaLajin* after childbirth?

Yes. *PaidaLajin* helps with insomnia, milk production, postpartum depression, and painful swelling of the breasts. It also helps a woman get back in shape. By practicing *PaidaLajin*, the mother can avoid medication, which is beneficial to the baby.

Is *PaidaLajin* suitable for a patient with osteoporosis?

Yes. *PaidaLajin* is excellent for osteoporosis. The main symptoms of osteoporosis are calcium deficiency and waist and leg pain. It is more evident in older people. It results from the blockage of multiple meridians. By practicing *PaidaLajin*, various nutrients will reach the entire body, healing osteoporosis. Adjust the duration and intensity to the patient's specific condition and tolerance.

Can sport and other traumatic injuries be self-healed?

Yes. In fact, *PaidaLajin* was initially used to treat traumatic injuries in Ancient China. As long as there are no fractures or open, bleeding wounds, you can *Paida* at and around the area. It relieves sprains, lumbar muscle strain, and muscle and tendon injuries. If *Paida* on the specific area is too painful, *Paida* pain spots at the corresponding area across the other side of the body. For example, your left elbow matches your right knee, your right ankle corresponds to your left wrist, and your left shoulder matches your right groin.

Gradually increase the intensity. *Paida* one area for at least fifteen to thirty minutes. To self-heal a severe injury, fresh or old, you may need to *Paida* several times. Stretching on a *Lajin* bench can help relieve almost all waist and leg pain.

Can skin diseases be self-healed?

Yes. Eczema, psoriasis, urticarial (hives), neurodermitis, allergic dermatitis, mosquito, and insect bites are symptoms. The root causes lie in the internal organs. Please reference skin diseases in the illnesses chapter for more information.

Can I self-heal dental problems?

Yes. *Paida* can help with toothaches, gum disease, mouth sores, loose teeth, tooth decay, tooth erosion, and sensitive teeth. You can slap regularly on the cheeks, mouth, chin, and the *Hegu* Acupoints on the back of your hands. Do *Lajin* on a bench as well.

Can I fix bad breath with *PaidaLajin*?

Yes. Bad breath tells us something is wrong with our internal organs, typically disharmony between the spleen and stomach. You can practice *Lajin* on a bench with sandbags on each leg. Slap the universal regions (elbows, knees, hands, and feet), and then along your four limbs for twenty minutes per part.

Can tinnitus, hearing loss, and deafness be self-healed?

Yes. Tinnitus, hearing loss, and deafness caused by injury, antibiotics, and old age are all related to blockages in meridians corresponding to the ears. You can slap at and around the ears and all over your head. There are a lot of hearing-related nerves and meridians on the head. In addition, slap the universal regions (elbows, knees, hands, and feet), and particularly along the inner side of each leg where the Kidney Meridian is located. Practice *Lajin* on a bench to enhance your kidney energy. According to Chinese Medicine, the Kidney opens to the ears.

Why do I have so much body odor during *Paida*?

Seriously ill patients, especially those under long-term infusion and medication, often emit various odors during *Paida*. This includes the smell of drugs, pesticides, and other chemicals. The smells of sweat, urine, and stool can be stronger. Their colors might be darker than usual. These are all healing reactions; drugs and other toxins are being expelled from the body. Continue *PaidaLajin* to further detoxify.

After slapping for forty minutes, there are cracks, white powder, and bluish-purple marks on my hands. Can I wash my hands now? Should I continue slapping, or wait until they have faded?

These healing reactions are good detoxification. It's best not to wash large cracks right away. Use warm water to wash them two hours after *Paida*. It is OK to continue *Paida*, even if they bleed a bit. With persistent *Paida*, the colors and powder will fade away, and the cracks will heal naturally. Your skin will gradually become smooth and delicate. Most of our coaches, and many *Paida* enthusiasts, have repeatedly experienced it. Their skin and overall health are getting better and better.

Why do blood blisters develop on my palms when I slap others?

When you use your hands to slap others, your hands are being slapped as well. It is a win-win situation. Blood blisters on the palms are healing reactions, indicating blockages in the Heart and Pericardium Meridians. Continue to slap. The blisters will break. Blood and fluid will seep out, and the wound and heart disease will heal naturally.

When stretching on the *Lajin* bench, why do I feel excruciating pain on the sides of the knees and near my groin?

This is typical. Pain indicates meridian blockages. Continue stretching and slap the pain spots, and you will gradually relieve the pain and self-heal your diseases.

Why do I sweat a lot during *PaidaLajin*?

Sweating during *PaidaLajin* is a healing reaction. The exercises boost the body's *yang* and clears waste through the skin pores. The self-healing mechanism regulates how much a person will sweat. After sweating, drink ginger and jujube tea to replenish your *qi* and blood.

Why has my body become so sensitive after *PaidaLajin*?

I sweat easily and avoid cold. Being sensitive to temperature is a desirable result. It shows some meridian blockages have been removed, and your body's immunity is being enhanced.

Some people are not sensitive to cold air, food, drinks, or water. They may even think, "The more, the better." These people accumulate a lot of cold and dampness in their bodies. An overreaction to heat implies your body is internally cold, and it is unable to clear it from your meridians. Sensitivity to cold is a good warning sign that cold is damaging your health.

Is it OK to practice *PaidaLajin* at night?

It's best to practice *PaidaLajin* in the daytime. However, some people only have spare time after a day's work or study. It's OK to practice it in the evening or night.

Do *PaidaLajin* immediately when experiencing strokes, fevers, coughing, headaches, itchiness, nausea, vomiting, stomachaches, muscle cramps, heart discomfort, breathing difficulty, menstrual pain, gall bladder pain, and other serious situations. Please read the section for acute symptoms for more information.

What should I do when family members and neighbors do not like the "noise" of *Paida*?

Paida does produce sounds. It can be too loud and annoying for people who do not yet understand and appreciate it. *Paida* when you're alone if necessary. Find an appropriate location to *Paida* with others who practice it. You can use your fists or tools to reduce the sounds, which we call "music."

When the time is right, and people are ready, explain *Paida* them to join you. Respect their decision either way. Many people will initially have doubts, and it's their business to change their own minds. You should never push *Paida* on anyone else.

Why does ginger and jujube tea make me nauseous? Why do I keep burping while I drink it?

If there is too much cold in your body, and the tea boosts *yang*, it is like fire melting ice. When you drink the tea, the positive and negative energies engage in a tug-of-war fight. Burping is a good reaction, because cold and foul air is being expelled. After your body becomes more balanced, you will appreciate the smell, taste, and function of the tea.

Can I drink ginger and jujube tea in the morning on an empty stomach? Can I drink it year-round?

Yes. You can drink the tea at any time of a day, and in any season. It's good to drink the tea while practicing *PaidaLajin*.

Most people have too much cold in their bodies, so make it a regular drink. It is best to have during the day. You can have some at night, but too much might cause insomnia.

Is vegetarian food good for health?

Yes. You can make rice, wheat, or other grains (that are nearly neutral in nature) your staple foods. Avoid cold air, food, and drinks, and too many fruits and raw vegetables. It can aggravate your conditions and cause new health problems. Many nutrient-rich foods are hard to digest if they are cold in nature, so you won't absorb the nutrition.

Can I reduce the dosage or stop taking medicine when practicing *PaidaLajin*?

It is up to your doctor. We are not doctors, and we do not provide any medical advice. Many people have self-healed their diseases by practicing *PaidaLajin* and have gradually reduced or stopped medication. However, consult with your doctor before making changes.

Do I need to go for regular health checkups?

It is up to you. Health screening is meaningful, but we recommend avoiding over-diagnosis and over-treatment. Some health problems can't be detected, and others can create unnecessary psychological burdens. You can do your own research on the subject.

In effect, *PaidaLajin* is a great way to check whether a person is healthy or not. Disease names are ignored, and *PaidaLajin* reveals if the meridians are blocked or not. As long as there is *sha*, pain, redness, swelling, or other reactions, there are meridian blockages and the person is sick. Diagnosis and self-healing happen at the same time.

Can you give me a more detailed self-healing regime?

There are no fixed rules. It differs from person to person. The duration, intensity, and frequency all depend on you.

Normally, whatever your health condition is: practice *Lajin* on a bench, *Paida* the universal regions (elbows, knees, hands, and feet), and slap along the four limbs, head and face, and then carpet bomb the body. You can also do meditation, wall hitting, waist swirling, and tie qiang gong exercises. We recommend drinking ginger and jujube tea and eating cooked, warm vegetarian food, primarily grains. Do not eat too much. Fast when you are ready for it. Avoid cold food and drinks.

TESTIMONIALS

I: *Paida* Saved a Dizzy, Hypertensive Patient on a Train

"The day before yesterday I took the High-Speed Rail G60 from my hometown Ningbo city back to Beijing. On the way, I suddenly heard an announcement—a passenger in Compartment Number Five was feeling some discomforts and needed a doctor or a medical professional's assistance.

Apparently, no one responded to this announcement. When I heard the same broadcast the fourth time, I stood up and went over to have a look. Well, I did not know what gave me the courage. I thought to myself, 'The passenger may be having cardiovascular disease or gastrointestinal disease. *Paida* might be of some help.' I felt a bit uncertain, although I was quite sure of the effect of *Paida*.

I arrived there and saw some attendants. They assumed that I was a doctor and were very happy I had come to offer help.

I told them, 'I am not a doctor. But I have some medical knowledge.'

They told me that the passenger was suffering from dizziness and hypertension. Hearing this, I felt more certain that I could handle it. They found a blood pressure meter and asked if I could measure blood pressure. I used to do it for my father. So, I told them, 'Yes.'

Soon, they moved the patient over to me. He was a man in his 40's or 50's.

The attendants told me, 'We have called for an ambulance. We will let him get off at the next station to receive first aid. There are over twenty minutes left. Please help relieve his symptoms.'

The patient's eyes were half closed, and he was frowning. He said he felt very dizzy. The attendants let him sit down and they looked at me, gesturing for me to measure his blood pressure. Seeing his condition, I felt that the top priority was not to measure his blood pressure, but to actually lower it. And the most convenient way to lower blood pressure is to slap on the inner elbows and *Neiguan* Acupoints. I put down the meter, took his left arm, and began to slap on the inner elbow. I asked an attendant beside me to help slap his right elbow. She hesitated, but then began to slap along with me.

The patient told me, 'I have high blood pressure. A few days ago, I went to a hospital in Ningbo and my readings were 130–150. I am going to Beijing for further examination and treatment. I did not take anti-hypertensive drugs this afternoon.'

While doing *Paida*, I told him, 'Just relax. *Paida* is similar to acupuncture and skin-scraping therapies. It will relieve your symptoms very soon.'

After a while, some *sha* appeared on his elbow. Then I moved on to slap his *Neiguan* Acupoints. The attendant did not slap hard for fear it would hurt the patient.

About five to ten minutes later, the patient was able to open his eyes. He said much of the dizziness was gone. He gestured for me to stop *Paida* and said, 'Thank you.'

The attendants were relieved to see his improvement. They said, 'The ambulance is waiting at the next station.'

The patient hesitated, 'I may not need it any more. I want to go to Beijing.'

However, the attendants still urged him to get off at the next station to receive first aid.

I went back to my seat in Compartment Number Four just next door. After a while, the train arrived at the station. The attendants arranged for the patient to get off the train.

Paida works really fast. I'm glad that I had the courage to offer him help. And I feel it a pity that most people do not know that simple *Paida* can help prevent and self-heal diseases; or perhaps, even if they know *Paida*, they do not take this simple folk therapy seriously. Well, in that case, the only option is to go to the hospital."

By Dear Natural Life
October 10, 2014
Original Chinese testimonial: 火车上的急救

II: *Paida* Healed a Three-Year-Old with High-Fever Induced Convulsions

"One day, I took my son to a small shop to buy things. When he was picking his favorite cookies, the owner of the shop suddenly cried out. It scared me, because I thought there was a robbery. I followed the sounds and found that his three-year-old grandson was in a coma due to high fever-induced convulsion, and the child's eyes were rolled upward.

I did not hesitate to think, but instantly grabbed his arm and began to slap on his inner elbow. The shop owner knew I could do pediatric massage, so he just let me slap him. One, two, three slaps ... as I continued *Paida*, the kid began to regain consciousness. I asked the shop owner to imitate me and slap his other arm. We slapped together for a while. Soon the child was conscious of the pain of *Paida* and tried to avoid it. But he was still not completely awake, and there were tears at the corners of his eyes.

I slapped along the arm to *Neiguan* Acupoints. Several dark spots of *sha* appeared at the slapped area. I slapped harder at *Neiguan* Acupoints. Suddenly the child burst into tears. Great! He was awake. What great joy!

Because I had learned pediatric massage, I knew his high fever-induced convulsions were caused by retention of food in his stomach. I asked the shop owner to give the child a massage on the abdomen in a clockwise direction. I also gave him a massage for bringing down his fever and relaxing his bowels.

The second day, when I visited the shop again, I saw the little boy alive and kicking. Had he been sent to the hospital, he would have been given several days of infusions. Moreover, it is hard to bring down a fever without harming indigestion. A doctor of Western Medicine may not have seen the root cause and would not have treated it holistically.

I'm glad that I know and practice the *PaidaLajin* self-healing method."

By Rui *qi*, from Xi'an, China
June 11, 2014
Original Chinese testimonial: 拍打急救高温惊厥幼儿

III: Paida on Breasts

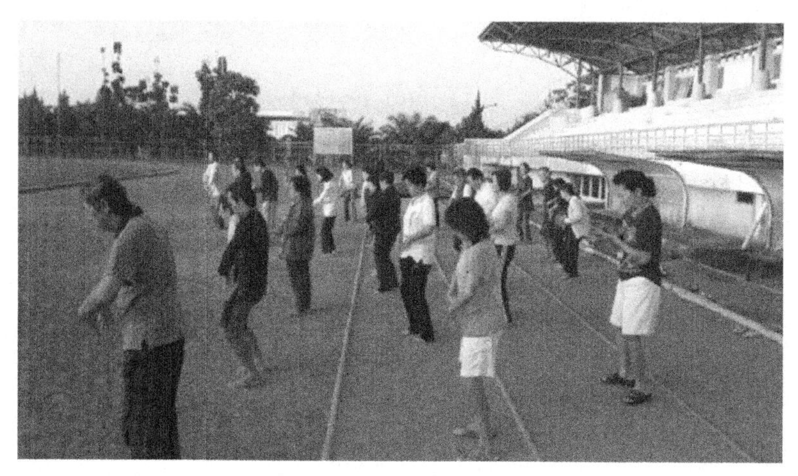

Anonymous (Chinese mainland)

"I think *Paida* on the breasts is a must for women. I have done it many times myself. This time I have recorded the whole process, and I'm eager to share it with others. If you do a random survey, you will find that virtually every woman has period pain and/or breast problems, such as soreness, swelling, and hard lumps. But it would be really foolish if she ignored these symptoms until they got out of hand.

In my case, at the beginning, my right arm felt sore and sometimes weak. I slapped it many times, but the soreness persisted just near my armpit. One day, my best girlfriend came over to help. Thanks to her heavy *Paida*, *sha* came out quickly. As I fully appreciated the health benefits of *Paida*, I did not mind the pain. All I wanted was thorough detoxification.

It's strange that *sha* emerged from where *Paida* wasn't the hardest, so she traced the *sha* and continued *Paida*. Then we found more bluish lumps toward my breast.

After half an hour, we traced *sha* down to the end, and I finally found that the problem was with my right breast. With the rhythmic *Paida* sounds, this kind of 'self-torture' really made me excited, for normally a woman's breasts do not get such heavy *Paida*. Thinking of one of my relatives, a forty-five-year-old woman, who lost half of one breast in a surgery, and many other women who have breast problems, I had to try very hard to clear the meridians around my breast.

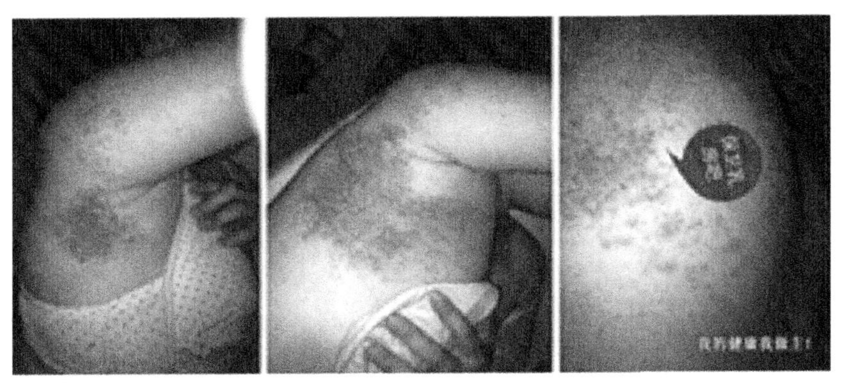

For the health of breasts. My health, I manage!

It lasted over one hour. My friend was tired. Bluish lumps were all over my right breast, and the red *sha* appearing in the beginning around my armpit had faded. *Paida* on my sore arm revealed that my real problem was with my breast. I felt so happy even though my skin and muscles hurt. Practice has proved that the human body is wise and will guide us if we listen to it.

In a few days, my period came again, and it was smooth, without any pain. My right arm, quite sore for years even if I slapped it a few times, is no longer sore after this round of *Paida*.

I am going to have my other breast slapped in a few days. A woman can never afford to be careless about her breasts."

My Comment:

In regard to breast diseases, women have the final word. There are many similar self-healing stories posted at my Chinese blog, including one special case where an egg-sized breast tumor disappeared after persistent *Paida*.

Dear women readers, more self-healing stories and photos are welcome (you may choose to remain anonymous.) This will help half of the world's population to relieve their agonies. And if wives and moms are healthy, won't their husbands and children be happy?

Original Chinese testimonial: 乳房拍打记录和照片

IV: Testimonials from the Soweto Nursing Home in South Africa

The following are some of the testimonials from elderly women at the Soweto Nursing Home in South Africa. For more testimonials from them, read "*Paida* and *Lajin* at an Old Age Home in South Africa."

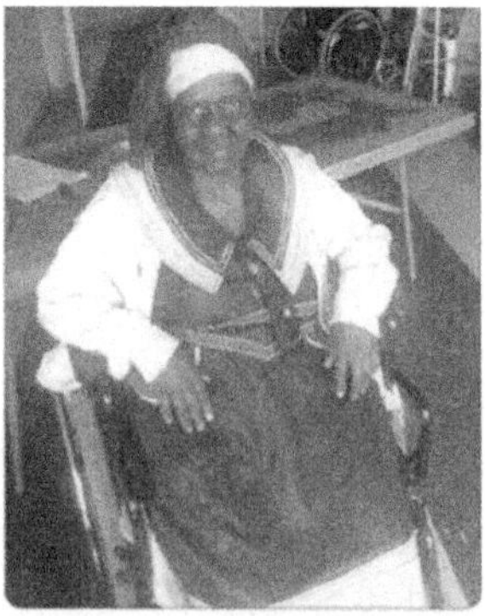

NAME: Ms. B. Nkosi
AGE: Seventy-two-years old

"I think coming to the Soweto Old Age Home was a blessing in disguise for me, because otherwise I would have never met Tshidi and Axel, who introduced me to *Paida* and *Lajin*.

I have diabetes and I'd had a stroke. My left side was completely dead, and I could not speak. But now I am a different person. I can speak and join in when others sing in church. I am regaining feeling.

It is a bit painful, but at least I feel something and am confident that soon I will be out of my wheelchair. I am truly grateful that Master Hongchi Xiao developed this life-saving technique and to Tshidi for devoting her time to help us. May the Good Lord bless all of you."

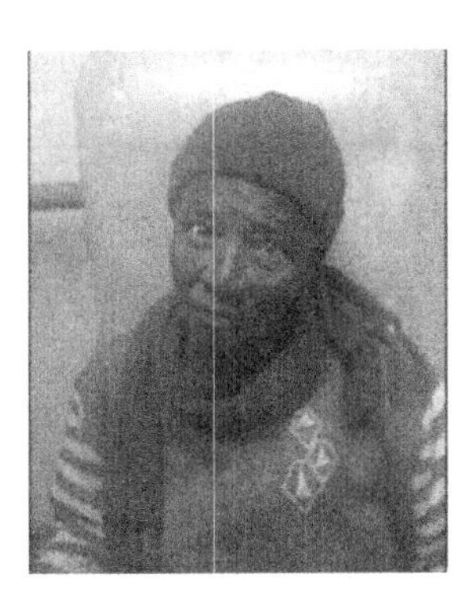

NAME: Ms. A. Skati
AGE: 83 years old

"I have been a diabetic and have suffered from hypertension ever since I can remember. My health has never been good. My legs and feet suddenly turn black and get painful at times. But ever since I started *Paida* and *Lajin* with Tshidi in September 2012, my health has improved.

My blood pressure is now normal when I go for check-ups. As for my diabetes, I can't even remember the last time I took insulin. I am grateful to Tshidi, Axel, and Master Hongchi Xiao for giving me my life back."

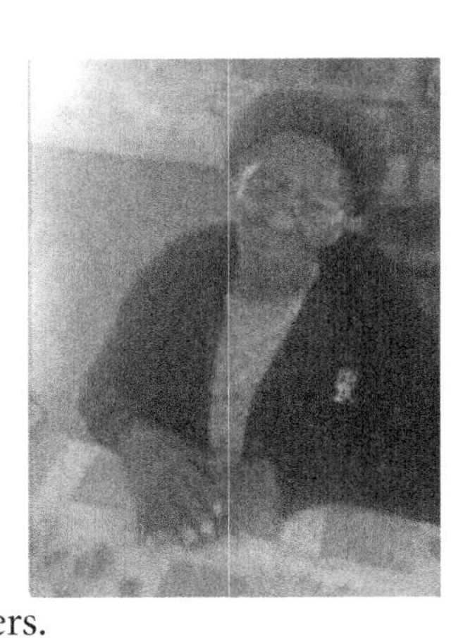

NAME: Ms. M. Mohai
AGE: Eighty-seven years old

"My body was aching so much that the painkillers were not helping anymore. This arthritis had stolen the joy of life from me. I had become partially blind, and that meant I had to rely on other people to help me with every little thing in life. To me that was frustrating, because I did not want to spend my golden years as a burden to others.

I was about to give up when Tshidi and Axel came into my life with Master Hongchi Xiao's magical *Paida* and *Lajin*. I am telling you I am a brand-new person now. I am back to going to church by myself every Sunday, going for a walk in the sun, and also doing a little work in my vegetable garden. I could not have done this without *Paida* and *Lajin*.

Thank you all so much."

V: Spine and Knee Pain Healed; Quit Smoking During Workshop

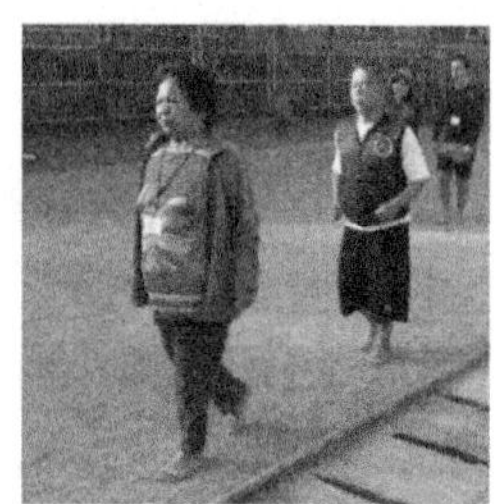

Pintolina: Sixty-five years old,
height 5'8", weight 156.5 pounds,
lives in Medan, Indonesia

"In October 2013, my mother was hospitalized in Columbia, Asia because of complaints in her spine and the knee joints resulting in severe pain when walking. MRI examination results showed that there was a pinched nerve in her lumbar sections L3, L4, and L5 of her spine, and osteoarthritis in her knee joints (right knee at stage 3 and left knee at stage 1.)

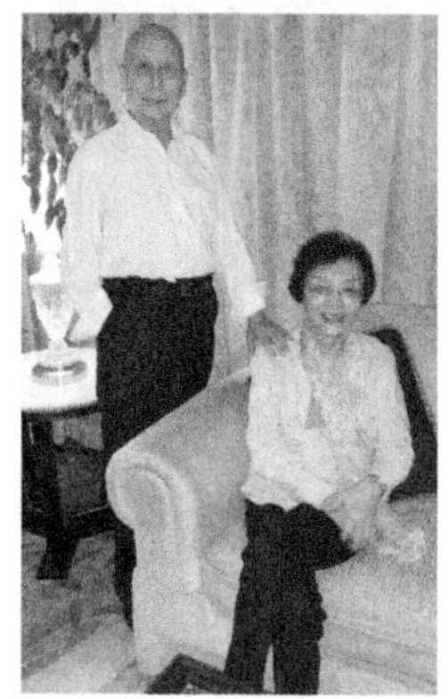

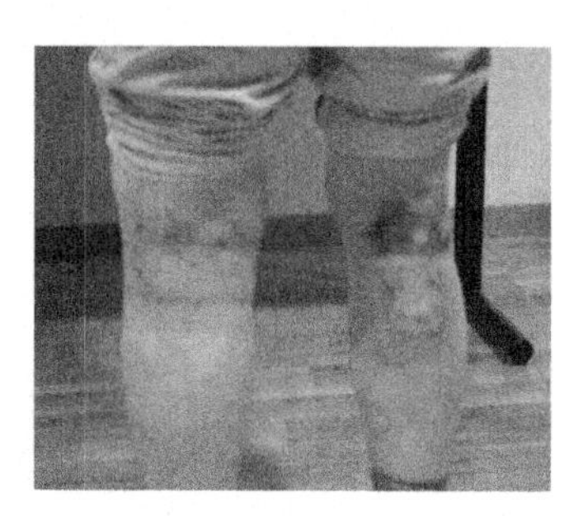

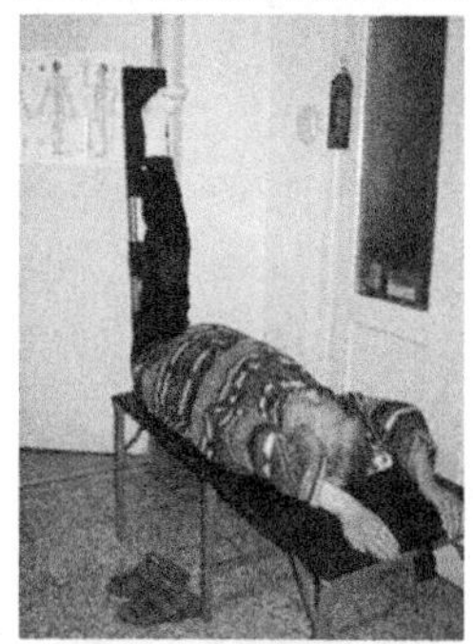

The doctors decided that surgery must be done immediately at the pinched nerves in the spine and then the next month knee replacement surgery (total knee replacement/TKR) in the right knee and steroid injection in the left knee. However, considering the financial factors and also the age factor (then sixty-three years old), my family decided not to operate.

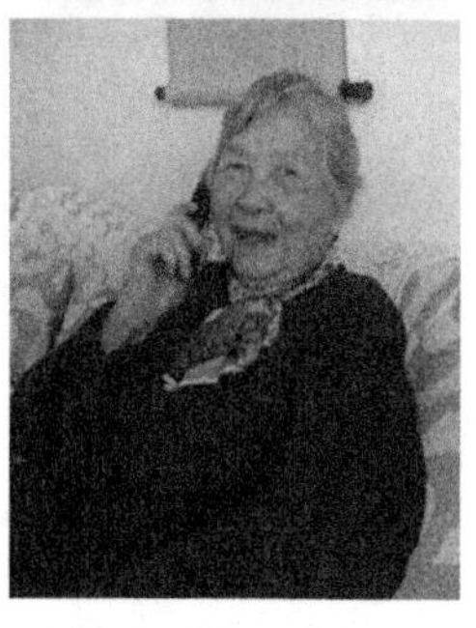

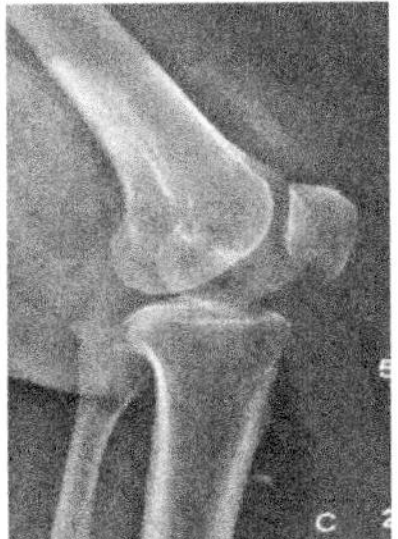
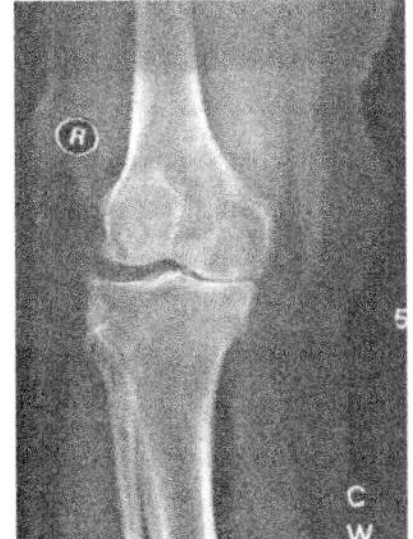
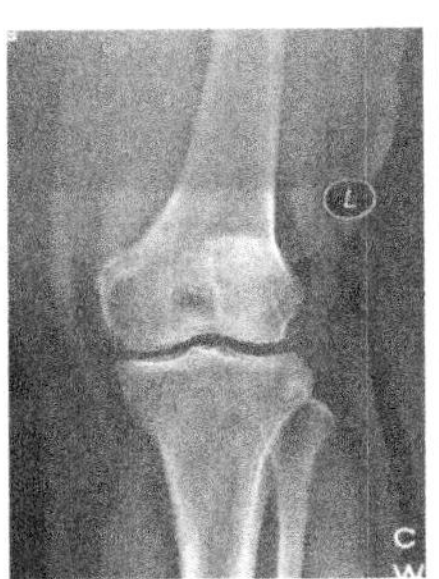
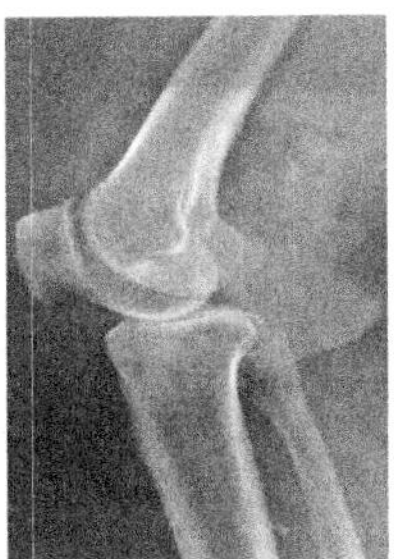
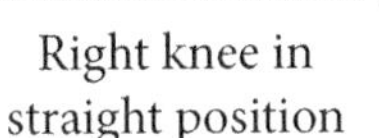

Right knee in straight position | Left knee in straight position | Right knee in bending position | Left knee in bending position

With conditions such as her legs and spine pain, my mother always took painkillers and other bone drugs (at least ten items of medicines) every day in order to walk and reduce pain in her bones. Other treatments were massage every two weeks and physiotherapy treatments.

My mother became familiar with massage treatment and physiotherapy, but the pain was still there. In November 2014, she switched to acupuncture treatment, but it was not very successful. The acupuncturist also suggested surgery, because according to him acupuncture could only help reduce the pain but would not fix the pinched nerve and bones that had osteoarthritis.

With the help of drugs, my mother endured the pain until March 2015, when she had to be hospitalized again. Her stomach lining had eroded and was virtually leaking (ultrasound examination results.) Most likely it was because of too many drugs over many years. Not able to stand my mother's suffering, I surrendered and asked for surgery on her knee.

Because of my mother's insistence, I started looking for information on recommended hospitals and doctors who conducted TKR in Medan, Jakarta, Malaysia, Singapore, and Thailand.

While looking for the information, one of my friends introduced me to *PaidaLajin* and sent me a YouTube link and an English manual. From the link, I looked for more information and became acquainted with Mr. Wong and Mr. Hanafi. I then joined a WhatsApp group to exchange information. The first impression that made me fall in love with *PaidaLajin* was that *PaidaLajin* information does not suggest taking drugs or supplements, and does not sell products, unlike other alternatives that eventually try to sell (multi-level marketing.)

I am very confident with the concepts of self-healing and "my health, I manage." I immediately applied *PaidaLajin* to my mother on April 26, 2015 and she stopped taking all kinds of drugs. The first week she did *Lajin* for twenty minutes on each leg with 4.5 pounds on her lowered foot, routinely every morning and afternoon. The eighth day (May 2, 2015) I did *Paida* on both of her knee joints, the backs of her feet, both inner elbows, and her entire back. Wherever I slapped, there was *sha*.

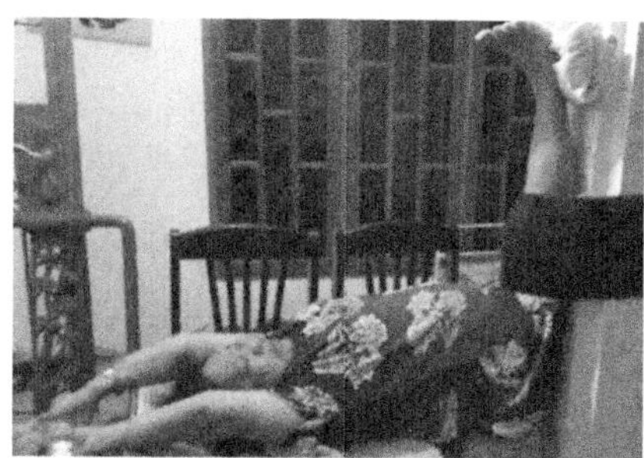

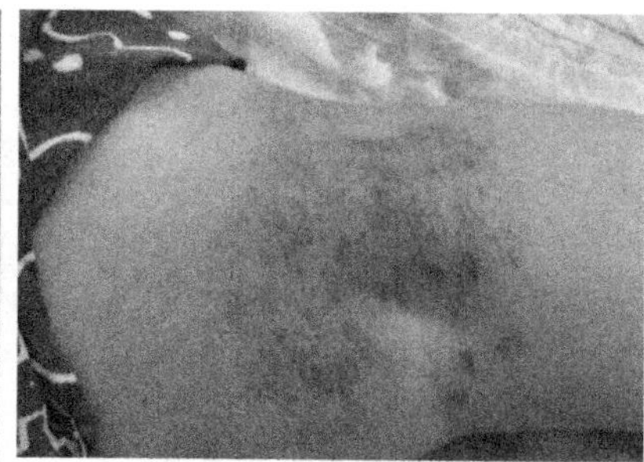

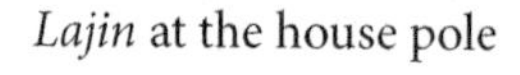

Lajin at the house pole

Paida on the knee

Beginning on the ninth day (May 3, 2015), my mother had chills and a fever for three days. *Paida* activity was stopped, but *Lajin* in the morning and evening continued for twenty-five minutes per leg, using nine pounds.

After the fever was cured, a week later on May 10, 2015, we again applied *Paida* on her calves, thighs, and underarms. But the next morning her chills and high fever came back, and my mother was sicker than the first time (healing crises, i.e., healing reactions.) I always shared how my mother felt in the WhatsApp group and was always guided online by Mr. Hanafi, Mr. Wong, Mrs. Ut, and the other group members. There was this incredible atmosphere of mutual support and encouragement, although we had never met personally. The second healing crisis was very painful. She not only had a fever; some parts of her body suddenly got swollen and then self-healed without treatment. Strange ...

During the week, fever and swollen left and right insteps alternately made my mother discouraged and unwilling to continue with *PaidaLajin*. At that time, I also panicked, and I had mental pressure from my brothers, who did not agree with the treatment of *PaidaLajin*.

But thanks to motivation from group members and talks with me through direct phone calls, my mother was finally willing to do *PaidaLajin* again, with a slight feeling of doubt and fear that the next healing crisis would happen again.

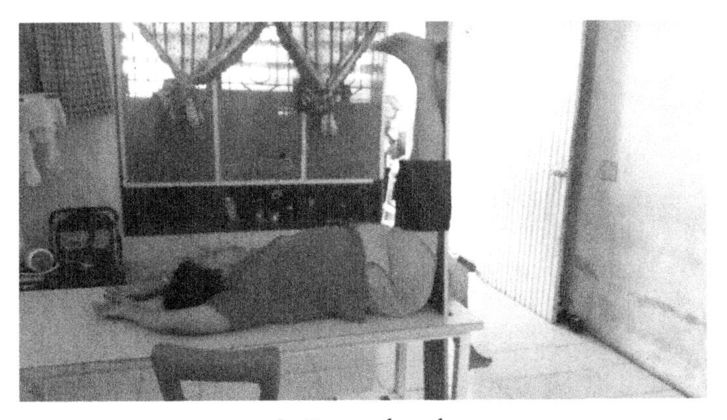

Lajin on a bench

Although I had not been convinced that *PaidaLajin* could heal my mother, I was determined to take my mother to Jakarta to meet with Mr. Hongchi Xiao and attend the seminar, *PaidaLajin* Self-Healing, in Jakarta on June 27, 2015. After the seminar, my mother and I finally decided to join the workshop in Bandung on June 29–July 5, 2015.

Feeling the money we invested in these activities was very large (in our financial condition), my mother and I did it seriously and sincerely.

My mother's health progress during the workshop in Bandung:

The first day:

My mother arrived with a stick and had to be guided to walk. After the initial examination, we followed a series of activities without the slightest complaint regarding the activities and the food menu "without rice, side dishes, or vegetables." We tried to accept sincerely that everything practiced in the workshop was the best for us. *PaidaLajin*, meditation, and sharing activities went smoothly that day.

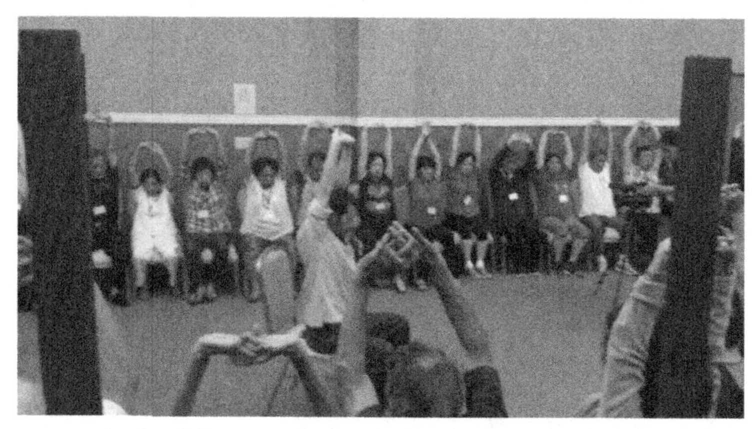

Workshop in Jakarta, Indonesida, July 27, 2015

The second day:

Jogging in the morning was painful for my mother. She was only able to walk about fifty-five yards while the other participants jogged around the field. Meditation was also a new thing for my mother. She sat there, but just to see other people meditate. After being given an explanation of meditation, she understood the benefit and decided to meditate more seriously the next day. *Lajin* was not difficult for my mother because she often did it at home, but *Paida* made my mother fear that the healing crisis would come again.

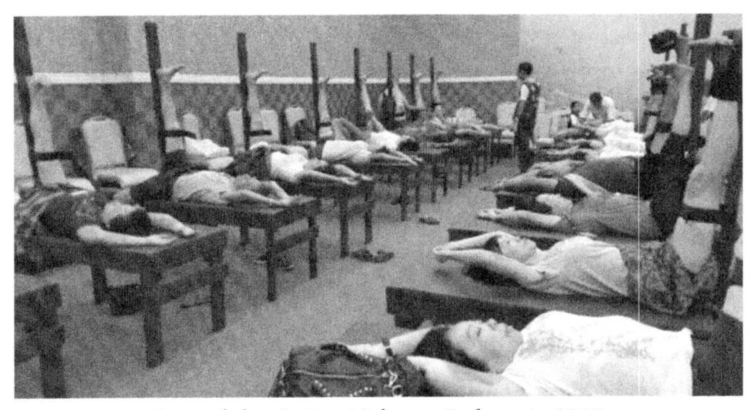

Second day *Lajin* at Jakarta, Indonesia 2015

The third day:

With extraordinary zeal in the morning, my mother was able to go two rounds around the soccer field although she rested eight times. On this third day, my mother was not using the cane anymore, but was still led because of her fear of falling. She followed *Paida* (carpet bombing) and *Lajin* with passion. She was much more spirited than when doing *Paida* at home, because of the group *Paida* atmosphere and mutual motivation in the workshop.

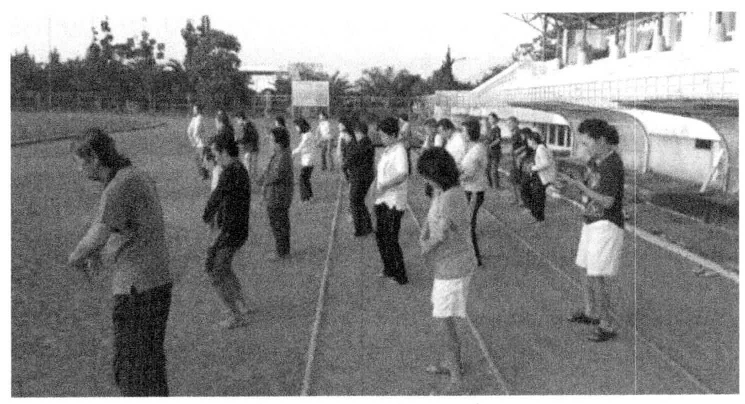

Third day waist swirling and jogging

The fourth day:

My mother was able to walk and jog four times around the field. Amazing! I was very happy to see my mother's health progress day by day. She had no painful healing crisis, was in much better health, and she felt more energetic although we began fasting on the fourth day. There was only ginger and jujube tea, but her body was more refreshed and energetic. Initially we were worried about her stomach disease, but strangely she felt no pain in her stomach during fasting. Fantastic.

The fifth day:

My mother jogged for five rounds in the soccer field without a break and without any complaints. Knowing my mother's progress, I was very happy and cheerful. Today she did *Paida* with more passion. My mother also testified to the workshop participants about how she felt.

The sixth day:

She was feeling pain in her legs only at the time she started to stand up. After standing up, five rounds around the soccer field was not a tough job for her. Jogging today felt light. All activities felt short today. Breakfast and her health examination were carried out at the end of the event.

Fantastic results: blood pressure of 145/86 down to 110/77, weight reduced from 164 pounds to 158 pounds, blood sugar dropped from 5.2 to 4.5.

One more result was no less important: my mother managed to quit smoking during the workshop. For decades, she had tried to quit smoking but failed. During the workshop, my mother felt very uncomfortable around the smell of cigarettes, and even inhaling cigarette smoke felt uncomfortable.

The seventh day:

She kept up her spirits and went jogging today, although some participants had already gone back home. We felt the sadness of separation from other participants who had become friends, mingled with a feeling of immense pleasure because of the health improvements achieved. Photo shooting and submission of testimonials turned into something very touching, and it was fun to hear the experience of peer participants during the workshop. My mother shared that she had imagined *PaidaLajin* would apply to family members and friends who were sick. Incredible! *PaidaLajin* is great for us who have financial difficulties, because doctors and hospitals are very expensive. My mother excitedly sang a song at the end of the workshop.

Changes in lifestyle and living habits have delivered a better life to my mother. It's too bad we didn't know about *PaidaLajin* sooner, but for a better life, there are no regrets. Just do it and you will have a better life.

My mother still jogs 1.25 miles every morning, does meditation, *Paida* and *Lajin*, and maintains her diet. She practices a simple and healthy lifestyle. Pain in her spine and knees and stomach disease disappeared after attending the workshop.

"Now I feel fifteen years younger than my age. I feel I am fifty. Fantastic!" said my mother.

Thank you, Master Hongchi Xiao, Master Hanafi, Master Wong, Master Kemal, and other masters of *PaidaLajin*. May we all enjoy a better life."

Personal experience: Pintolina
Written by Simson, Pintolina's son
Posting by *paidalajin*indo@gmail.com

VI: *Paida* Healed an Eighty-Six-Year-Old Patient with Terminal Prostate Cancer

My Comment:

Many people assume that patients with terminal cancer and weak *qi* and blood can't practice *PaidaLajin*. What revelation does this testimonial give us? Of course, we can't conclude that all terminal cancer patients can go through such heavy, thorough *Paida*, but it is OK to start *PaidaLajin* gently, and then gradually increase the time and force. *PaidaLajin* can be for everyone.

When diagnosed with prostate cancer the first time, Eva's father already had his testis swollen for more than ten years, to as big as the size of two eggs, in addition to having difficulties when he urinated. But after only three *Paida* sessions, these symptoms all disappeared, including his prostate cancer. However, Eva's father feared the pain of *PaidaLajin*, so he did not sustain the effort. In June 2014, he was diagnosed with terminal prostate cancer.

From Eva's story, we can tell her father did not suffer from just prostate disease, but from complex diseases. But as terminal prostate cancer was most deadly; it became the foremost problem. Eva's father went through four months of bone removal, radiotherapy, and other conventional therapies, but was only left with near-hopeless results. He was meant to be saved by *PaidaLajin*. With much *yin* came the rise of *yang*—Eva's experience of self-healing rheumatoid arthritis and her unmovable confidence in *PaidaLajin* gave her great strength to help slap her father and heal him. It took her 4.5 hours just to slap one leg, and he was in pain and groaning the whole time. After nearly three months, his prostate cancer was gone, and his prostate gland was in better shape than some middle-aged men. And almost all his other diseases were gone too.

Eva's father did not do *Lajin*. Had he practiced *Lajin*, he would have recovered faster. Eva's sharing also includes some key takeaways that will benefit all readers. We are grateful to Eva and his father for making miracles happen.

"Dear Mr. Xiao,
Hello!

I am still feeling too excited to calm down. And I do not know where to begin telling you this.

I still remember in mid-June 2014; my father's legs were in so much pain that he could not walk. We took him to the hospital and went through a series of check-ups, including scans, x-rays, ultrasound, blood tests, urine tests, and puncture tests (twelve punctures.) The results indicated that my father had terminal prostate cancer. His prostate specific antigen (PSA) level was at 25 (PSA is a diagnostic indicator for prostate cancer. Normally, a no-cancer PSA reading should be less than 4.) My father's cancer had spread all over his body, the malignant tumor was two inches big, and even his hip bone was already fractured and infected with cancer cells, requiring immediate steel-plate internal fixation. When our family heard this news, we felt like the sky was falling down. It was very sad for us to know that our father, who was very intolerant of pain, had to go through the torture of cancer in the last days of his life.

In order to understand my father's condition more thoroughly and get more expert advice, my family and I went to visit another three urologists. They all confirmed my father's condition was as what the hospital had diagnosed. They all told us, 'There is no way your father's cancer can be completely cured, because it is already at the terminal stage. The cancer cells have already spread to his head and all over his body. The most that can be done is to give him some shots, surgically remove parts of his bones that got 'eaten' by cancer cells and add steel plates to them, go through radiotherapy, and remove his testicles. These therapies might somewhat extend his lifespan, and allow him to have dim sum (a local Hong Kong dish) close by.

At that time, my eighty-six-year old father's condition:

1. He could not walk and needed to move around in a wheelchair; he could not even put his feet onto the wheelchair footplate. And he needed to be moved onto and off the bed.
2. Could not even turn over his body in bed.
3. Always needed to use a urinal.
4. Had no appetite.
5. High blood pressure.

6. Had prostatic hypertrophy; he needed to urinate quickly and frequently, it was painful, and he could not completely empty his bladder. His urine came out weak and in spurts. Night urination increased, and he had to urinate every twenty to thirty minutes at night.
7. Constipation. He had to take laxatives.
8. Extreme pain in his shoulders, arms, back, waist, buttocks, legs, and knees.
9. Low white blood cell count and platelet count (anemia.)
10. Weak kidneys.
11. Cold hands and feet: had to wear woolen socks and turn on the heater even in the summer.
12. Calves and the bottom of his feet were numb.
13. Legs turned blackish, all his toenails were infected with fungi, and both his feet were completely hardened with dead skin.
14. Both feet were swollen to the point where we could not see his ankles. His right calf (the one that needed steel plate surgery) was so swollen that it turned transparent, and hard as a rock.
15. Cancer spread to his chest and his chest bones protruded, which could be seen easily.
16. He fainted very often.

My father experienced the typical symptoms of terminal prostate cancer, like swollen testicles and the clogging of urine. In 2013, when my father was first diagnosed with prostate cancer, his testicles were swollen to the size of two eggs. They had been swollen for more than ten years, and he had been taking medicine for more than ten years. But not only had he not experienced any improvements, his condition got worse. He had tried other folk methods too, like applying ice to his testicles, and blowing them with a blow dryer—but still no improvements.

One day he could not urinate and feared that this might become uremia, so he went to see the doctor. That was when it was first discovered that he had prostate cancer. The doctor immediately referred my father to another hospital for treatment.

My mother has always believed in *PaidaLajin*, and persuaded my father by saying, "Let your daughter help you *Paida*. Only *Paida* can save you now." My father didn't go to the hospital, and came home to let me *Paida* him. I had *Paida*-ed him three times, each for over two hours, only at his groin and on his stomach. His testicles have not swollen up since, and there is no more clogging when he urinates either.

The doctor checked my father's condition one month later, and told us that he had recovered from prostate cancer. Now, this diagnosis seems overly hasty and simple, and my elderly father did not know how to ask for the details and diagnostic factors. Hearing the doctor say 'recovered,' he left the hospital feeling happy. As my father could not bear the pain, he did not continue *Paida* to clear all meridian blockages. This might be why his prostate cancer relapsed. Even with just three *Paida* sessions, the benefits were still significant—my father still hasn't experienced the swelling and clogging.

In June 2014, when my father's second PSA reading came out to only 25, even the doctor was in doubt. Based on how serious the spread of cancer was at that time, my father's PSA reading should be at least in the hundreds or thousands. The doctor even wondered if prostate cancer was not the origin of his cancer, and had my father go through a very detailed check up again, but the results were the same. Only our family could explain this. After all, I had slapped my father two years ago, which may result in interesting body reactions that others may not be able to comprehend.

On July 22, 2014, my father went through a surgery to remove cancer-infected bones, and they connected his bones with plates. On July 31, he was given a hormone shot to relieve pain. On August 26, he was given one session of radiotherapy. During this time, I sought advice from the radiology departments of two private hospitals; both responded that each major pain area had to go through at least ten radiotherapy sessions. I have a friend who had prostate cancer with no metastasis, had to go through radiotherapy at the most renowned private hospital in Hong Kong for five times a week, and spent HK$300,000 [about $38,000 USD] in a month.

All of the doctors said my father's condition would improve after these treatments, and his pain would much subside. At that time, my father wished very much that he would see big improvements, but unfortunately, that did not happen. Even though he could walk with crutches, and could occasionally limp without them, his condition fluctuated a lot. One week he was better, the next week he got worse, and he needed to take larger and stronger dosage of painkillers, which could barely hold down his pain for twenty-four hours. What was swollen became even more swollen, and stiffer, like a piece of iron. The skin on his legs started to lump like cucumber skin. His skin turned blacker, like there were worms inside, chewing on his legs. He always fainted, and a few songs kept ringing in his ears again and again. He could not sleep and was very frustrated.

After almost four months of conventional therapies, the diagnostic report on October 9 indicated a PSA reading of 21, just 4 readings better, which was a disappointment. By then my father had lost all hope, and wanted to give up on all treatments, and thought of leaving the world early rather than keep on suffering. Oh ... the saddest thing in this world is when there is no way out in living, but you can't choose to die. You have absolutely no choice in anything.

Whenever you feel you have lost all hope, or when the whole world—including doctors and specialists—all discourage you by saying, "irreversible", "there is no hope", "this can't be cured", and "you will never get cured," please, you must remember Mr. Xiao's dictum: "Ignore the disease name. All illnesses are due to blockages of the meridians. Unblocking the meridians heals." These words of wisdom gave me and my family immense confidence and encouragement, so I begged my father, "Please let me help you with *Paida*."

My father had not let me slap him, because he was too fearful of the *Paida* pain, but then he had no other choice. On the afternoon of October 7, I started *Paida* my father for the first time after he was diagnosed with terminal prostate cancer. I slapped him with both of my hands, starting from his groin down to his legs, for at least ten minutes each spot, down to the back of his feet, then to the inner and outer sides of his feet, and the soles of his feet. Since my father was very weak, almost no *sha* came out. In spite of this, I still patiently slapped him in a carpet-bombing way. I slapped 4.5 hours for each of his legs, and he was in great pain and groaned for 4.5 hours. I had to stop.

The second day, my father told me his leg pain had subsided a little and he felt better. The third day, he told me his legs had been very itchy the night before, and he scratched them and could feel there were fluid coming out, but the blackish color of his legs was lighter. The lumps of his skin also smoothed. These were the miraculous benefits of just one *Paida* session. We had to continue with this battle, didn't we?

On the third day and the fifth day, I slapped my father again. I slapped him every other day. Except for the first week when I slapped him three times, for the weeks to come, I slapped him twice a week, four hours each time. It was not because I did not want to *Paida* him more, but he was in fear of the pain. He did not let me *Paida* him more. I very much wanted to *Paida* him every day, so he would heal faster.

After every *Paida* session, there were immediate, significant improvements to my father's health condition. Sometimes even before the *Paida* session had completed, the benefits were already there. For example:

1. Initially his arms were in so much pain they could not be lifted, but after one hour of *Paida*, he could lift them.
2. After *Paida*, he could pull his arms backwards, which he had not been able to do before *Paida*.
3. When I slapped his stomach, his constipation was immediately relieved, and he had to rush to the bathroom to release his bowels.
4. His legs used to be in so much pain he could hardly walk. After *Paida* he felt much lighter when he walked.
5. After I slapped his head just once, the repeated songs in his head almost stopped, and only some faraway tunes were occasionally heard.
6. After six sessions of *Paida* in twenty-one days, the bone protrusion in his chest flattened.

On October 29, the hospital report indicated normal white blood cell and platelet counts, with no signs of anemia and normal kidney function. New bones grew too after surgery, and most importantly, his PSA reading went down to 0.2 (a normal reading is less than 4.) This indicated no more cancer cells existed, and my father's condition was even better than an average man's. The doctor was so happy for my father and congratulated him.

I was honest with the doctor and told him *Paida* healed my father. The doctor encouraged us, 'Then you should continue *Paida* on your father. For now, he does not need any more check-ups or therapies from the hospital. All we need to do is to keep monitoring your father's condition.'

This report result was so encouraging, confirming what Mr. Xiao had told me, "*Paida* is the best, purest, most natural, and organic form of chemical therapy." Isn't that right? Other than being rid of all cancer cells, other usual terminal cancer readings including white blood cell and platelet counts, anemia, and weak kidney functions, all went back to normal very quickly. The self-healing power was fully mobilized to combat cancer, and at the same time cleared toxins from the body, healing new and old diseases altogether, not only clearing the symptoms but also diseases from its sources, turning back the aging clock—all for free.

Conventional radiotherapy and chemotherapy not only kills cancer cells but also normal cells, have huge side effects, and result in pain and discomfort that can be as severe as what a patient suffers from cancer. Moreover, these therapies are expensive. We know all these facts.

During this time, we invited our parents and other family members for two vacations. My father enjoyed himself like a normal person—he could eat, jog, play, and sleep. He walked a few hours at a time and did not need to go to the bathroom all the time either. For twenty-plus years, he had experienced difficulties whenever he had walked more than ten minutes. He was overweight and had degenerated knees. Back then, his doctor had advised him to do knee replacement surgery. Luckily, he rejected that advice. He walks normally now.

January 6, 2015 was the day when my father was to undergo testis removal surgery, as arranged by the hospital months before. On January 3 (five more days to go to make it three months of *Paida*), we wanted to check my father's condition again. We did not dare to hope that his cancer was all gone; we would be happy if the tumor had shrunk. The ultrasound test results were: normal (no tumor), no signs of testis swelling, and a slight swelling of the prostate gland. (The doctor said my father's prostate gland condition was extremely good considering he was eighty-seven; it would be unfair to compare his condition with a schoolboy.) Residual urine was at 23 c.c., which was better than for an average middle-aged man. Before the ultrasound test, my father had drunk more than ten cups of water, but had no need to urinate until two hours later. His bladder capacity was at 300 c.c.—which was again—given his age, considered extremely good. A typical prostate cancer patient could have ultrasound tests without having any prior fluid intake, as he would already have a swollen prostate gland and testis.

Based on the test results, the doctor told us, "Everything is normal. Even better than a healthy fifty-year-old man." He even asked me, "Did you or the hospital make a mistake? It is impossible that your father is a prostate cancer patient. There must be a mistake."

After we saw this most wonderful report, we called the hospital to cancel the scheduled testis removal surgery, and we informed the hospital that my father no longer had the tumor and there was no need for surgery.

But the hospital did not believe it. How could that be possible? The tumor was so big. It could not just disappear. The doctor had made it very clear. The removal of testis in a prostate cancer patient with no metastasis might cause the tumor to shrink, and hopefully, the patient would be able to live with his tumor. But after such surgery, many would experience urinary incontinence, and would need to use adult diapers.

I secretly giggled at such responses. Nobody believed this miracle. But in the world of *PaidaLajin*, miracles happen every day. We are used to it, and only outsiders can't comprehend this. *PaidaLajin* empowers everyone to self-heal diseases; even for complicated diseases it is very simple. It all depends on your faith, will, and action.

My father's conditions explained earlier are all healed, except for some residual toenail fungi and some dead skin on his feet. His face now shines. He has two bowls of rice at every meal and walks freely. He is full of energy and has no need to take any medicine. My mother, being kind of jealous, jokes to me, "Your father's health is better than mine now—you need to *Paida* me too."

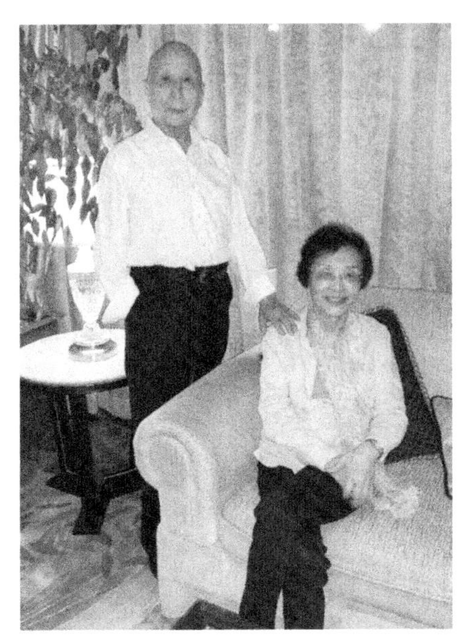

Father and Mother Happy Together

From diagnosis to the thorough cure of terminal prostate cancer, my father had not taken any Chinese Medicine, done *Lajin*, taken chemotherapy, lost his testis, or had a tumor removed. He only received *Paida*.

I wish to briefly share some tips about my father's *Paida* again:

1. *Paida* as closely to the prostate gland as possible (no *Paida* on the penis and testicles.) Then *Paida* outward, at least ten minutes on each area. *Paida* around the anus too, with the help of a *Paida* stick.

2. *Paida* longer where there is pain. *Paida* is a way to combat pain with pain. I started *Paida* with both of my hands at first, and after seeing *sha* appear, I would *Paida* the same area using a *Paida* stick with more force.

3. Areas I always slapped: I started *Paida* heavily on the heart area with both of my hands for twenty minutes. Then I moved onto the lungs, then to the stomach, and then to the start of

the thighs, for about ten minutes each. If I did not have enough time, I would slap each area for five minutes. This way, the heart, liver, spleen, stomach, kidneys, and intestines would all be covered. Mr. Xiao often reminds us, "If the heart is well, all will be well; if the heart is not well, nothing will be well." For other body parts, I took turns slapping them, and eventually the whole body went through a thorough *Paida*.

4. You need to be patient and not rush. *Paida* can be gradual, from soft to heavy, and there should definitely not be any moving-around-here-and-there *Paida*.

5. Suggestion: For a very sick patient, *Paida* should be done every day, and for longer time periods; this will enable faster healing.

Mr. Xiao, thank you again. We are now able to enjoy good health only because of your unconditional promotion of *PaidaLajin*."

With much gratitude,
By Eva Ka
Email: keva198@gmail.com
January 16, 2015
Original Chinese testimonial: 86岁晚期前列腺癌痊愈记
*You can visit our websites to read Eva's father's test results.

VII: How to *sha*ke Off Doubts and the Doctor's "Spell"

"My mom has been doing *PaidaLajin* for nearly two years. She is eighty-eight and quite healthy. Even when she occasionally feels uncomfortable due to slight hypertension, gastric acid, or occasional constipation, she relieves the symptoms through the earnest practice of *PaidaLajin*. During the past two years, she has had—by turns—doubts and confidence in *PaidaLajin*. As she is an 'intellectual,' naturally, she quite often demands scientific explanations. If she is not satisfied with the answer, she will regard it as unscientific and harbor doubts about it.

The height of 'war' with mom came after she had been practicing *PaidaLajin* for nearly a year. At the time, her health had dramatically improved. After stopping all medication, her heart condition and blood pressure remained stable, years of dull pain in her stomach disappeared, the pain in her joints was relieved, her constipation and insomnia were greatly alleviated, and her neck problem was cured. But then, mom decided to do a thorough check up, saying, 'I need scientific proof that I am indeed healthy.'

Prior to that, whenever mom went to the hospital, she had to take a cab. Her heart could not stand the discomfort of public transport, and she could not walk that far; but surprisingly, when she went for the check-up, she took a bus there along with her caregiver (we call her Auntie.) When having her blood pressure measured, she thought she must have high readings after such a torturous bus ride. But to her surprise, the readings were 120/80. It wasn't even that good when she had been taking antihypertensive drugs. Mom was very pleased.

Two days later, the blood test results came back. All the indicators were normal, except for slightly high blood fat. When the doctor asked her what drugs she was taking to control the levels, Mom replied, 'Nothing.'

The doctor overwhelmed her with criticism and 'what is scientific'. Because mom had two coronary stents (a heart surgery), the doctor warned that without taking lipid-lowering drugs, there would be life-threatening danger. But what the doctor chose to ignore—or was simply not interested in—was the fact she had normal blood pressure and all other indicators were good without medication for more than a year. In the end, mom took home a pile of 'life-saving drugs'.

I would call home each day. Knowing she was having doubts again, I tried to explain that the goal of *PaidaLajin* was to remedy all disharmonies in her body, including high cholesterol. Anyway, a slightly high level in a single indicator did not mean much. But mom was determined to work along both lines, because the doctor had warned that her life would be in danger if she did not take the drugs.

She asked me, 'Why are you so against medication? Why can't I take the drugs and do *PaidaLajin* at the same time?'

In fact, I had explained it to her time and again. And over the past few decades, the piles of costly drugs had not cured her of anything. Instead, she had gained new diseases due to the side effects of medication, and she had gotten weaker and weaker as a result of higher dosages and intake of more varieties. *PaidaLajin* activates the self-healing power in us, while medication tends to suppress and damage it. The so-called 'working along both lines' approach is useless. However, having been brainwashed by the doctor, Mom hastened to the dead end without turning back. And her voice went higher and higher when arguing with me. I had to let it go, even when tormented by much anxiety, due to fear that her blood pressure would go up if she got too excited. I had to respect her choice, and leave it to fate.

I was sleepless that night, a rare thing for me. I deeply felt that it may be easy for children to have filial affection, but how hard it is to effectively perform filial duties. The next day, with a very disturbed mind, I phoned Mom as usual. I was ready to let go of my insistence, for after all, the self-healing methods only cure diseases, and are not responsible for life and death. To my surprise, Mom did not use the same high-pitched voice she had the day before, and strangely spoke in a soft tone.

Just as I was wondering why, I heard her say, 'I'm stretching now.'

I asked her jokingly, just like when I was a mischievous child, 'Why are you still stretching? Don't the drugs solve it all?'

Then I heard Auntie's loud laughter and Mom had to confess. After my last call, she dared not take all the drugs as prescribed, so she swallowed only one hypolipidemic tablet (for lowering blood lipid levels.) Then she had a severe headache and later stomach cramps. She was tortured by the pain and relieved it with *Paida*.

She told me, 'Now I finally realize what you meant when you said working along both lines would not work.'

Facts speak louder than words. From that day on, Mom has shaken off the doctor's 'spell.' She gained a new and deeper insight into the self-healing methods, and has firmer confidence in them.

One year has passed since then, and mom has given up on medication altogether for up to two years. She only practices *PaidaLajin*, and her condition is very stable. During the period, she has not even had a bad cold, which shows her immunity has remarkably improved. This is the stable and fundamental source of her health.

For more than two years, I have been practicing *PaidaLajin* myself and have shared it with over 100 people. I have genuinely felt the power of one's mind and heart in the treatment of disease. One's thoughts inevitably impact the results. The best efficacy of *PaidaLajin* can be achieved only with harmony and oneness of the body and mind. Oneness refers not only to harmony of the body and mind when one is doing *PaidaLajin* himself, but also to the giver's and receiver's state of mind when helping each other *Paida*.

Recently, I have been receiving calls and emails from readers anxiously asking for my advice on how to help their sick parents. They face the same dilemma I did. Their parents tried *PaidaLajin* in order not to disappoint them, but deep down, they did not really believe in it. When they experienced healing reactions, or when they did not see instant improvement, they would have doubts and give up, or choose to go to the hospital.

Here is my advice. Ask yourself honestly, 'How much confidence do I have in *PaidaLajin*?'

If you have full confidence in it, I believe you will find your own ways to influence and lead your loved ones to continue and gradually build their confidence through practice. It is only a matter of time and patience. If your family can't accept them, then let it go, because if the giver and receiver are not of the same mind, it will not yield good results. If you yourself lack confidence, then I suggest you practice what you advocate in the first place.

Our thoughts play a decisive role in our lives and in our health. And they can be changed. When we shake off our doubts, we will enhance our physical and mental wellbeing."

"Righteousness keeps away evil."

"Mindfulness keeps away evil thoughts."

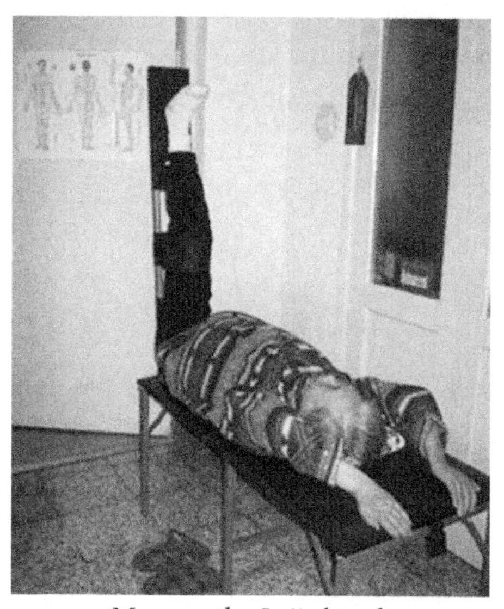

Mom on the *Lajin* bench

By Fei Schmitz
April 15, 2012
Original Chinese testimonial:
如何摆脱疑惑和'医咒'—— 读李晶博文后有感

My Comment:

Fei Schmitz's mother has turned ninety. She used to take 42.5 tablets a time, three times a day. She has taken no medicine for years after practicing *PaidaLajin*. She slaps and stretches every day and is enviably healthy. Fei Schmitz has become a *PaidaLajin* promoter, based in Germany.

Email: info@*lajin-paida*-deutschland.com
Website: www.*lajin-paida*-deutschland.com
Facebook: facebook.com/*lajinpaida*deutschland
Twitter: KunstdesDao

Consider a thirty-nine-year-old hypertensive patient, Mr. Huang Changsheng, from Malaysia; a muscle atrophy and rheumatoid arthritis patient, Eva, from Hong Kong; and a diabetic patient, Mr. *Yang* Weijie, from Macau. They all applied *PaidaLajin* immediately, signed up for a workshop, and persisted after they returned home. Their confidence, determination, and perseverance healed them.

Mr. Huang Changsheng, humiliated by his family, stood firm when they criticized *PaidaLajin*. Mr. Huang healed his hypertension without medicine, and eventually his wife and daughter used *PaidaLajin* to heal themselves. Then his family turned their house into a *PaidaLajin* center. Dozens of people learn in this center.

When Eva had lost all hope, at the height of *yin* came the rise of *yang*. Eva's immense determination was activated. She did *PaidaLajin* for ten hours a day. This paid off. Her muscle atrophy, rheumatoid arthritis, and other diseases were all healed. Later on, she slapped her father, helping heal his terminal prostate cancer and other illnesses. She is now a *Paida* expert.

Mr. *Yang* Weijie had taken so many insulin shots his stomach had rotted. Other than diabetes, he also had diseases of his heart, liver, and kidneys. After attending a workshop, he no longer needed medication or insulin. It's been four years, and all his medical tests still come out normal. He is now a professional slapper who helps others to heal themselves.

ABOUT THE AUTHOR

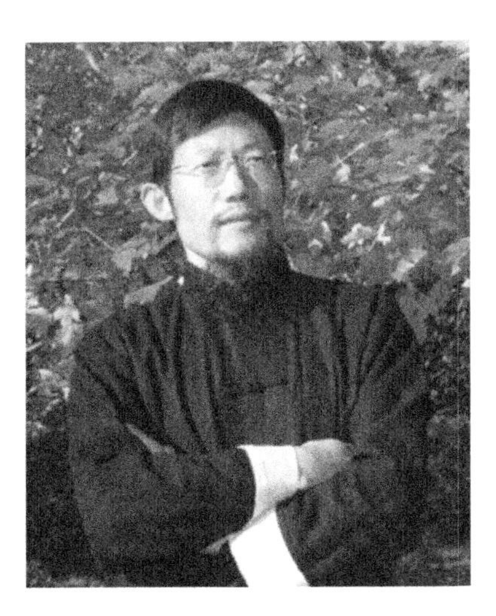

Mr. Hongchi Xiao was born in Hubei Province, China, and is dedicated to promoting the *PaidaLajin* self-healing method worldwide.

In 1990, Xiao got his MBA and subsequently worked in the finance area in the US and Hong Kong for over a decade. Though he had a comfortable life in the business world, Xiao often felt a lack of purpose in life. Starting in 2000, he began to trace his roots of Chinese wisdom. In 2006, he met a monk who told him he was destined to study at some temples and monasteries in the mountains of China.

For the next few years, Xiao followed the list mapped out by the monk and studied with healers, Taoists, monks, and hermits. This series of events led him to rediscover Chinese culture and to learn, from masters of Classical Chinese Medicine (CCM), many therapies previously thought lost, including *Paida*, *Lajin*, acupressure, acupuncture, bone setting, and needle-knife.

Then he began his healing journey in Tibet, where he healed a few thousand people for free. After that, he opened a clinic in Beijing. At this clinic, he asked patients waiting for treatment to practice *Paida* (clapping and slapping) and *Lajin*, a special form of stretching. Many people relieved their symptoms simply through *Paida* and *Lajin*, before even seeing him for treatment. Suddenly this 'healing by oneself' concept overtook him.

Since then, Xiao has been dedicated to promoting these treasures, particularly the simplest ones—*Paida* and *Lajin*. While the other therapies do work wonders, they are nonetheless quite complex and are still a passive means of 'healing by others'. They are not safe, simple, and effective methods of healing oneself, and therefore can't be easily affordable and accessible to all.

Xiao believes we are our own best doctors. To promote this lifestyle and to empower people to self-heal, Xiao has authored such best sellers as *Journey to Self-Healing* and *PaidaLajin Self-Healing*. Now he is traveling the world giving lectures, organizing workshops, and demonstrating *PaidaLajin* to promote self-healing. He has visited scores of Chinese cities, India, Indonesia, Singapore, Malaysia, Australia, Britain, France, Germany, Switzerland, Bulgaria, Holland, Canada, the US, South Africa, and Lesotho, to name a few. New calls will take him to places, big or small, when conditions are 'ripe'.

Xiao asks doubters and theorists: "Have you tried *PaidaLajin*?" For Xiao and the millions who have benefited, the only way to test the efficacy of *PaidaLajin* is to JUST DO IT!

Join our global self-healing movement

English website: www.pailala.org (with 105 video lessons)
English Facebook: www.facebook.com/*PaidaLajin*Global
English YouTube: Journey to Self-Healing
English website: www.*paidalajin*.com/en/

Chinese website: www.*paidalajin*.com
Chinese blog: blog.sina.com.cn/yixingtx
Chinese Facebook: www.facebook.com/*paidalajin*selfhealing
Chinese Wechat No.: *paidalajin*999

Deutsche website: www.*lajin-paida*-deutschland.com

***PaidaLajin* in other languages (download from www.pailala.org):**

Arabic
French
German
Indian લાજીન (in Gujarati) (in Marathi)
Indonesian
Japanese
Romana
Russian
Spanish
Thai

Available in perspective countries:

Bosnian
Bulgarian
Greek
Malaysian
Serbian

To purchase a book on Heart Chan Meditation:

"DeStress, Energize & Awaken Through Chan Meditation"
On Amazon: https://www.amazon.com/dp/1456466410/

To attend Heart Chan meditation classes in the USA:
www.heartchan.org

FINAL WORDS

The biggest challenge I've encountered since I began promoting *PaidaLajin* is the unbelievable nature of its healing power. Most people, when hearing my presentation, cannot believe these two simple techniques can heal almost all illnesses.

Though matrix biology has certified a system that connects all of the cells in our bodies, the pioneers of matrix biology have not tried *PaidaLajin* yet. Though based on Traditional Chinese Medicine, *PaidaLajin* improves microcirculation, but there is no instrument that can visualize the changes as deeply as the organ level. Microcirculation detection instruments can only function about a quarter of an inch deep.

Since there is no scientific or medical certification, and because its healing is almost miraculous, it's difficult to explain it to the media. Many bloggers, tabloid magazines, and news articles—in many countries—have questioned the method. How can I defend the reputation of *PaidaLajin*?

I hear case after case of healing coming from every corner of the world every day, and I'm humbled.

I want to defend this magnificent technique. Let's do it together.

There is some concern I'm trying to revolutionize the medical industry, but this is not the case. My goal is simply to complement current medical practices and for people to heal themselves first, under the supervision of medical professionals. Since the medical industry is slow to respond to new information, and people all over the world seek my experience, I cannot ignore the requests from people who suffer.

For *PaidaLajin* to become a massive self-healing practice, it requires an awakening in every one of us. It needs resources to promote it. It needs certification from the medical industry. And, most importantly, it needs to begin with every one of us. Please try it and witness it. Then, and only then, will you know if *PaidaLajin* works.

For now, my focus is simply to save everyone I can.

I've often been asked, "Why is it so effective? It's almost miraculous." My answer is often the same, "It is a gift from the God in all of us."

Practicing *PaidaLajin* is no different than any spiritual practice. The only way to witness God is to dedicate oneself completely. There is no need to listen to others, and need no permission from anyone else. It is a direct personal experience. A person must have faith without suspicion and truly surrender the ego.

The human body is not a random combination of elements. It was designed and manifested by a superb being with wisdom and love. Sometimes people have different names for this superb being, such as Spirit, God, or Dao. Although names vary across different cultures, it all points to the same ultimate source. Everything observed about *PaidaLajin* was witnessed gradually, naturally, and automatically through human practice. Human beings struggle to understand the intricate creation by God with their incomplete knowledge. Therefore, the more a person surrenders to God—to Dao—the easier it is for us to witness God's creation.

Simply put, *PaidaLajin*, the two simple mechanical movements, cannot produce healing directly. It simply switches on the self-healing system God pre-designed in us. The self-healing is achieved by automatic cellular information exchanges, biochemical reactions, and energy enhancement. Self-healing is like the key to a car. The simple action of turning the key can start the car, but the software and the hardware are manufactured and ready to go. The real instrument of self-healing is God. The distinguishing feature of self-healing is allowing God's creation to function as it should. The less human intervention, the more God's manifestation.

The self-healing method introduced in this book comes from Chinese Medicine, which is derived from Daoism. As a follower of

Chinese culture, I was neither close to, or distant from, God. I was in the status of half-believing and half-doubting. However, as a result of advocating and practicing self-healing all over the world, it made me a believer and worshipper of God. *PaidaLajin* kept making me ask, "Why?"

Both Chinese and Western Medicine use their own methods of discovering and explaining God's creation. Each has its own achievements and shortcomings. Both are limited in discovering and explaining the how, but not the why. Human exploration and discovery are an endless process. This is God's design. Facing the unknown, human being need more humbleness, surrender, and belief in The Creator.

Chinese calls this "Respecting the Dao and valuing morality." (*Dao De Jing*, Chapter 51). Here is a quote from the Bible: "In the beginning was the Word, and the Word was with God, and the Word was God." (John 1:1) Eastern's Dao and Western's God are one, just with different names. Self-healing made me find God, and God allowed me to find my life's purpose: that is to glorify God through advocating self-healing.

Now, let me come back to the most frequently asked question: "How can such a simple method achieve miraculous results? Why does such a simple method heal so many different kinds of disease?"

I can only say: "Amazing healing comes from God's amazing grace."

Therefore, the more you believe in God (Dao, The Creator), the more you will achieve! There is only one way to determine if my witness is true or not: everyone, including every doctor, hospital, and scientific research institute, please do your own clinical experiments first and then draw your own conclusions. Let us propagate this self healing movement.

All healing and all glory belong to God!

Hongchi Xiao
January, 2018
Australia

Printed in Great Britain
by Amazon

29846813R00165